Homelessness and ill health

Report of a working party of
the Royal College of Physicians

Edited by
James Connelly
June Crown

1994

ROYAL COLLEGE OF PHYSICIANS OF LONDON

Royal College of Physicians of London
11 St Andrews Place, London NW1 4LE

Registered Charity No. 210508
Copyright © 1994 Royal College of Physicians
ISBN 1 86016 009 3

Typeset by Oxprint Design, Aristotle Lane, Oxford OX2 6TR
Printed in Great Britain by The Lavenham Press Ltd,
Lavenham, Sudbury, Suffolk

Members of the Working Party on Homelessness and Ill Health

Sir Anthony Dawson KCVO MD FRCP *(Chairman)*

Dr J M Crown FRCP FFPHM *(Honorary Secretary)*
Director, South East Institute of Public Health, Tunbridge Wells, Kent

Dr H S Allinson BSc MB BCh
General Practitioner, Abingdon

Dr J B Connelly MRCPsych MFPHM
Senior Lecturer in Public Health Medicine, University of Leeds

Dr C C Evans MD FRCP
Consultant Physician, Royal Liverpool University Hospital

Mr K Judge MA PhD(Cantab)
Director, King's Fund Institute, London

Dr T J Lissauer FRCP
Consultant Paediatrician, St Mary's Hospital, London

Dr M Marshall MRCPsych
*Training Fellow, Unit for Research in Social and Community Psychiatry,
Warneford Hospital, Oxford*

Dr I M Murray-Lyon MD FRCP
Consultant Physician, Charing Cross Hospital, London

Ms B Shoderu MSc
King's Fund Institute

Mrs R Short HonMRCP
*Member of Parliament, 1964–1987; Chairman, Select Committee on Social
Services, 1979–1987*

Professor D R London DM FRCP
Registrar of the Royal College of Physicians

Dr D A Pyke CBE MD FRCP
Past Registrar of the Royal College of Physicians

Mrs S A Thewlis BA MIPM
Past Deputy Secretary of the Royal College of Physicians

Observer

Dr K Binysh DCH MSPHM
Department of Health

In attendance

Miss E Stephenson BA (*Working Party Secretary*)

Ms B Coles MA (*Working Party Secretary*)

Acknowledgements

The Royal College of Physicians Working Party on Homelessness and Ill Health was established on the initiative of the Past President, Professor Dame Margaret Turner-Warwick and we are grateful to her for encouraging the College to consider this important topic.

The Chairman and members of the Working Party are also most grateful to the following people who presented evidence to them and whose knowledge and experience were invaluable in developing ideas and recommendations:

Dr Isobel Allen, *Policy Studies Institute*

Mr Dominic Burn, *Shelter*

Professor Susan J Smith, *Department of Geography, University of Edinburgh*

Dr Christina Victor, *Department of Public Health Medicine, Parkside Health Authority,* now at *Department of Public Health Sciences, St George's Hospital Medical School*

Dr Fred Woodroffe, *formerly Consultant Physician, Highlands Hospital, London*

We thank Police Sergeant Geoffrey Woolgar and Police Constable Alan Sayers of Charing Cross Police, who generously shared their experience of the single homeless people in their area and made their local statistics available to us. We also thank Dr Paul Roderick for his help in developing ideas contained in this report.

Ms Barbara Coles, the Working Party Secretary, worked tirelessly to co-ordinate the group's activities and we wish to thank her most warmly for all her efforts.

Mrs Muriel Harding and Mrs Gill Robinson of the South East Institute of Public Health and Mrs Barbara Hayes of the Division of General Practice and Public Health Medicine, University of Leeds prepared and amended numerous drafts of this report, for which we are most grateful.

The College acknowledges with thanks the generous support of the Abbey National Charitable Trust Ltd for their grant towards the costs of the working party and the printing of this report.

Foreword

The Royal College of Physicians has a long tradition of concern for the factors which affect health, as well as for the treatment of disease. This report continues that tradition by drawing attention to the relationships between health and homelessness. The number of people who are homeless has risen sharply over the last decade and they are to be found in all parts of the country. Some of them become homeless because of ill health. Most of them experience deterioration in their health as a result of homelessness. Many have difficulty in obtaining appropriate medical care.

This problem can only be tackled by the concerted action of Government departments, local authorities and health authorities, with support from other agencies. The Royal College of Physicians urges these bodies to adopt the recommendations of this report in an effort to diminish the problems of people who are homeless now, and for future generations.

I would like to thank the Chairman of this Working Party, Sir Anthony Dawson, the editors of the report and all the Working Party members who gave much time and thought to this work. I believe they have made a major contribution to the debate on this important health issue.

November 1994   LESLIE TURNBERG
                                                    President
                                                    Royal College of Physicians

Contents

Appendices

List of Tables and Boxes

BOXES

General Summary

There are three main groups of homeless people. Only one group, mainly families with children or pregnant women (described in this report as Group I), are *officially* recognised as homeless. In 1992 there were 169,966 of these statutorily recognised homeless households in Britain.

Rough sleepers and direct-access hostel dwellers (described in this report as Group II) are *not* officially homeless and *not* included in official statistics. In the 1991 Census there were 2,827 rough sleepers and 19,417 hostel dwellers in Britain.

The third group comprises those who are sharing accommodation or are otherwise inadequately housed. As very little information exists about these people, this report concentrates on Groups I and II.

The types of housing that are available in Great Britain are: owner-occupied and private-rented, for both of which an adequate and reliable income is required; and local authority or housing association rented housing, together described as social-rented housing, where access is intended to be based on need rather than ability to pay.

Poor health and disability limit people's access to housing, because they often reduce employment opportunities and hence income, so home-ownership or private renting are out of reach. The social-rented sector has decreased considerably in size over the past few years, making access to it more difficult. The mechanisms intended to ensure that people in poor health have adequate housing (medical priority for rehousing) do not work effectively.

Homeless families (Group I) have been shown to experience more mental, physical and obstetric health problems than comparable housed groups. They make greater use of hospital and community services. This is probably related not only to their health problems but also to the difficulties they have in gaining access to primary care. For many of them, a 'healthy lifestyle' is unattainable in crowded accommodation with inadequate cooking and recreational facilities.

Single homeless people (Group II) have a higher risk of death and disease than comparable housed people. Excess deaths are due mainly to suicide, accidents and violence, and alcohol-related and respiratory diseases. Single homeless people are prone to a wide spectrum of physical illnesses, involving all bodily systems. Among the specific conditions common in this group are tuberculosis, chronic obstructive airways disease (bronchitis), foot problems, infestations and epilepsy. The physical vulnerability of single homeless people, together with problems of compliance with treatment, pose special problems in relation to tuberculosis, where drug resistance may emerge with potential public health implications.

Single homeless people are more likely to have serious mental illness than the general population. Schizophrenia is the most commonly diagnosed disorder. The effects of mental illness, together with associated social and economic problems, can precipitate housing crises which the individuals concerned are unable to resolve and they thus become homeless. Community care programmes developed by health and social services do not take adequate account of housing need and so are not able to deal with these problems.

Various initiatives have been introduced in an attempt to improve health care for homeless people. On the whole, although valuable, they are small-scale and unco-ordinated and have only a limited impact on these very considerable problems. Although the long-term goal is to provide homeless people with services that are integrated with those for the rest of the population, special arrangements are needed in the meantime for primary care, accident and emergency services, community care and discharge planning.

This report confirms the strong relationships between homelessness and health. **It recommends** that the Government, Local Authorities, the Housing Corporation and the NHS should, as a matter of urgency, develop a co-ordinated approach to the development of a housing and community care policy. This is seen as a prerequisite for progress in this field.

Since it is unlikely that there will be rapid, dramatic improvements in the underlying causes of homelessness, there should be short-term arrangements to improve access to health care for homeless people.

In addition, future official statistics should include single homeless people (Group II); there should be regular monitoring of the health of homeless people; and current research on health and homelessness should be extended.

Recommendations

TO GOVERNMENT

The report draws particular attention to the different, and sometimes unintentionally conflicting, policies of different agencies. We believe that considerable improvements could be achieved and resources more effectively deployed if there were better integration. The key recommendation is therefore:

RECOMMENDATION 2 (*Chapter 2, p 37*)

> The Government, Local Authorities, the Housing Corporation and the NHS should together undertake a wide-ranging review of housing and community care policies, addressing the opportunities for integration and the barriers to progress. The aim should be to develop a co-ordinated action plan which identifies and provides the organisational, management and resource requirements to allow the implementation and evaluation of a coherent joint policy.

It is not widely recognised that single homeless street and hostel dwellers (described as Group II homeless people in this report — see page 5) are not officially designated as homeless and are not included in Government statistics.

The **Department of the Environment** is therefore invited to adopt:

RECOMMENDATION 1 (*Chapter 1, page 27*)

> The statistics collected on homelessness should be expanded to include rough sleepers and hostel dwellers (Group II homeless people) and such people should be officially recognised as homeless.

The **Department of Health** is invited to adopt:

RECOMMENDATION 7 (*Chapter 7, page 108*)

> The Department of Health should introduce systematic monitoring of the health of homeless people and their access to services.

This should include:
- principal and secondary health problems
- ethnic mix
- age and sex
- HIV infection, subject to informed consent and prescreening counselling
- tuberculosis
- GP registration
- hospital admissions
- type of homelessness
- accommodation on discharge

The results of such monitoring should be published as a regular report.

RECOMMENDATION 8 (*Chapter 7, page 108*)

The NHS Research and Development Directorate should take a lead in commissioning further research on the causes and consequences of all types of homelessness, building on earlier studies.

RECOMMENDATION 9 (*Chapter 7, page 109*)

The Government, through the proposed Regional Offices of the NHS Executive, should take steps to ensure that homeless people are not disadvantaged because of the financial implications of their care for GP fundholders. Although capitation mechanisms should take this into account, in the shorter term, arrangements should be considered, which could:

i   organise the funding of special practices for homeless people in such a way that these practices would be allowed to administer their own budgets and hence compete with GP fundholders;

ii   restructure deprivation payments to GPs by including a per capita payment which incorporates an amount based on the number of homeless people registered at the practice;

iii   co-ordinate a nationwide service for handlng the medical records of homeless people, thus ensuring that information is transferred smoothly between practices;

iv   set national health targets relevant to the health needs of homeless people;

v   co-ordinate a national strategy to provide better health care to homeless people.

Such a strategy would permit homeless people to choose where they wish to receive care either from a non-fundholding practice, a fund-holding practice or a special practice.

TO HEALTH AUTHORITIES, FAMILY HEALTH SERVICE AUTHORITIES AND GENERAL PRACTICE FUND HOLDERS

The Report identifies the health problems of homeless people and their difficulties in gaining access to services. These should be specifically addressed, as set out in:

RECOMMENDATION 4 (*Chapter 3, page 47*)

Health commissioning authorities should assess the health and health care needs of members of homeless households and should commission services to meet these needs.

RECOMMENDATION 5 (*Chapter 3, page 47*)

Health Authorities and Family Health Service Authorities should ensure that members of homeless households placed in temporary accommodation have access to full registration with a local general practitioner.

JOINTLY TO LOCAL AUTHORITIES AND HEALTH AUTHORITIES

Many aspects of the care and support for homeless people require the joint action of Local Authorities and Health Authorities. These authorities are invited to adopt:

RECOMMENDATION 3 (*Chapter 2, page 38*)

Within the recommended joint policy (see Recommendation 2), the current medical prioritisation procedures should be reviewed and integrated with community care and housing need assessment procedures. The conferment of priority need status should not prevent the assessment of housing need in relation to health need.

RECOMMENDATION 6 (*Chapter 5, page 89*)

Within the wide-ranging policy review (see Recommendation 2)
  i Community care of severely mentally ill people requires full implementation of the Care Programme Approach and care management. Both should explicitly include adequate housing

as an essential component. Community care should be seen as a combination of appropriate care and appropriate housing.

ii Community care plans drawn up by local authorities should specify the housing requirements of severely mentally ill people. Central Government should ensure that resources are available for capital developments (buildings and renovation), rehabilitation and support.

iii Direct access hostels should not be expected to provide care for severely mentally ill people. Health care commissioning authorities should ensure that a range of community and in-patient services are accessible to such people, complemented by an adequate supply of suitable housing.

1 Definitions, statistics and context of homelessness

SUMMARY

Three groups of homeless people are identified:

Group I

- Statutorily accepted homeless people — mainly families with children or pregnant women.
- This group constitutes the *official* homeless, that is, those who are included in the official statistics for homelessness.
- In 1992, 169,966 households were statutorily homeless in Britain.

Group II

- Rough sleepers and hostel dwellers — mainly single men.
- This group is *not* statutorily homeless and *not* included in official statistics.
- In the 1991 census, 2,827 rough sleepers and 19,417 hostel and common lodging house dwellers were enumerated in Britain.

Group III

- Other groups with inadequate housing.
- There are no satisfactory statistics for this group, though a 1990 survey of sharers found 73,000 families in England sharing accommodation who said they strongly desired to live separately.

The housing supply comprises:
- Owner-occupied housing

1

- Private-rented housing
- Social-rented housing
  - local authority rented housing
  - housing association rented housing.

There is a severe shortage of affordable, social-rented housing. The annual output of local authority and housing association rented housing currently falls short of need by 70,000 dwellings in England alone.

INTRODUCTION

This report aims to define the relationships between homelessness and health. It looks both at the health problems that can lead to homelessness and at the health consequences of homelessness.

It is well known that an individual's health status is influenced by a combination of biological, socio-economic and behavioural factors.[1] Strategies to improve health have to take these factors into account, as has been recognised by the Government in its proposals relating to the health effects of public policy choices in the White Paper *The Health of the Nation*,[2] and in similar strategies produced for Wales, Scotland and Northern Ireland.[3–5] Such recognition is vital, because each individual can control only some of the complex personal and environmental factors that interact to affect health. Government and other social institutions must therefore endeavour to produce and implement policies that protect and promote health; arrangements to ensure that each citizen can obtain and live in decent housing are central to such policies.[6,7] The UK government is a signatory to the World Health Organisation's 'Health for All' strategy (Box 1) which identifies *adequate shelter* as a prerequisite for good health and within Target 24 sets objectives for the provision of 'healthy houses' for the European region.[6]

This publication brings together the scientific evidence on the relationship between homelessness and health. Although there are methodological problems in analysing this relationship,[7] the available evidence is considerable and increasing. It points consistently to the conclusion that homelessness is damaging to health.

We endorse the importance of sustained action to improve access to decent housing as a contribution to improving the population's health, while acknowledging the complex relationships between homelessness, housing need and factors such as unemployment and poverty.

BOX 1

Target 24: Human ecology and settlements
By the year 2000, cities, towns and rural communities throughout the Region should offer physical and social environments supportive to the health of their inhabitants.

This target can be achieved if intersectoral, ecological approaches combining community planning and public health are used to improve the built environment and if countries take action to:

• ensure active community participation in determining needs and problems, and in the processes of planning and action;

• adopt community planning approaches that emphasize ecological concerns and the needs of people, and facilitate social interaction in all human settlements;

• strengthen programmes for the construction of healthy houses and housing improvement, including proper sanitation facilities and the provision of open spaces and recreational areas;

• meet the needs of special groups such as young families, the old and people with disabilities;

• introduce measures for intersectoral action to mobilize the support and resources of all sectors in community improvement;

• reach agreement on international health criteria for community planning and development, including housing, management of domestic waste, noise control and safety, and strengthen legislative, administrative and technical measures and services.

Source: *Health for All: the health policy for Europe.* WHO Regional Office for Europe, Copenhagen: 1993. (Ref 6)

DEFINING HOMELESSNESS

Although there is no universally accepted definition of homelessness, we believe that it is possible to set out a satisfactory definition for describing relationships to health. Two approaches have been considered. The first is to locate homelessness along a spectrum of housing need. The second is simply to adopt a legal definition.[7,8] The arguments underlying these two approaches are different and need to be understood in order to avoid confusion.

A *spectrum of housing need* starts with rough sleeping on the streets, moves through various types of insecure and unsatisfactory accommodation to housing that, though secure, is not considered adequate by the dweller (Box 2).[8] There is no agreement about the

BOX 2

Spectrum of housing needs

- People literally without a roof over their heads including those regularly sleeping rough, newly arrived migrants, victims of fire, flood, severe harassment or violence, and others.
- People in accommodation specifically provided on a temporary basis to the homeless (hostels, bed and breakfast hotels, short-life housing, etc).
- People with insecure or impermanent tenures: this includes other ('self-referred') hotel or bed and breakfast residents, and those in holiday lets, those in tied accommodation who change job, tenants under notice to quit, squatters and licensed occupiers of short-life housing (eg short-hold secure tenancies) and owner-occupiers experiencing mortgage foreclosure.
- People shortly to be released from institutional accommodation, including prisons, detention centres, psychiatric hospitals, community or foster homes, and other hostels, who have no existing alternative suitable accommodation or suitable existing household to join.
- Households which are sharing accommodation involuntarily.
- Persons or groups living within existing households where either (i) relationships with the rest of the household, or (ii) living conditions, are highly unsatisfactory and intolerable for any extended period.
- Persons or groups living within existing households whose relationships and conditions are tolerable but where the individuals/groups concerned have a clear preference to live separately, also cases where the 'potential' household is currently split but would like to live together.

Source: *Homelessness and the London housing market.* School for Advanced Urban Studies, 1988. (Ref 8)

point on this spectrum which divides significant from insignificant housing need and thus defines homelessness. Evidence suggests, however, that to be useful for the study of relationships with health a definition of homelessness should encompass a broad rather than a narrow view.

The *legal definition of housing need,* as used for Government statistics, relies on criteria for formal acceptance of households as 'homeless'. Households that fulfil these criteria acquire certain statutory rights in relation to housing and constitute the 'official' homeless. In the UK, the 1977 Housing (Homeless Persons) Act (consolidated in Part III of the 1985 Housing Act) placed duties on local housing authorities to help homeless people. Box 3 shows the types of situation that constitute homelessness within the terms of the Act, and describes the groups of people who are granted 'priority need' status, for whom the local authority is obliged to secure permanent housing. At the time of writing (July 1994) the Government is considering wide-ranging changes to the homelessness legislation. These proposals and their likely effects on health and health care are discussed in Chapter 6. The operation of the current legislation, set out in Fig 1.1, shows that two additional criteria must be fulfilled. The applicant for housing must not be 'intentionally' homeless, and must have a 'local connection' to the local authority's area of responsibility. The 1985 Act recognised the responsibilities of the state in relation to housing, but the definitions it adopted exclude from official recognition many individuals and households with significant housing needs who thus do not benefit from the law. Single-person households, couples without dependent children and many rough sleepers are the main groups affected. They, with others, constitute the 'unofficial' or 'hidden' homeless.

Since there is no ideal definition of homelessness with which we can satisfactorily explore and describe the links with ill health, we have adopted *working definitions* which relate to those often used in epidemiological and clinical studies and which incorporate the notions of housing need and the prevailing legal definitions. Three groups of homeless people have been distinguished:

Group I   Statutorily accepted homeless individuals and households placed in temporary accommodation by local authorities. These are mainly families and pregnant women. *This group constitutes the 'official' homeless.*

Group II Rough sleepers, night shelter and direct-access hostel users, and self or agency (not local authority) referrals to bed and breakfast (B&B) hotels. *This group is mainly NOT included in official statistics.*

Group III All other groups in housing need (see page 17).

Gypsies and travellers are not considered in this report. Their health needs differ sufficiently from those of the three homeless groups to make comparisons appear forced. Elements of their lifestyle and inadequate NHS responses to it do, however, increase risks of ill health. The health and health care needs of gypsies and travellers have recently been documented.[9-12]

BOX 3

Definition of homelessness and categories of people who are potentially eligible for statutory rehousing

---

Definition of homelessness

Under the current law, local authorities are required to make enquiries where a person applies to them and they have reason to believe that that person may be homeless or threatened with homelessness. Applicants are considered to be homeless if:

• They have no accommodation they are entitled to occupy; or
• They have a home but are in danger of violence from someone living there, or it is not reasonable for them to continue to occupy it; or
• They are living in accommodation meant only for an emergency or crisis (for example, a nightshelter); or
• They are a family who are normally together but are now living in separate homes because they have nowhere to live together; or
• Their accommodation is movable (for example, a caravan or houseboat) and they have nowhere to place it; or
• They have accommodation but it is not reasonable to continue to occupy it.

People are considered as being threatened with homelessness if they are likely to come into any of the above categories within 28 days.

Priority need categories

• People who have dependent children;
• Pregnant women;
• People who are homeless because of a fire, flood or similar emergency;
• People who are vulnerable because of:
  – old age;
  – mental illness or handicap;
  – physical disability; or
  – other special reasons

Source: *Housing the homeless: the local authority role*. London: Audit Commission, 1989. (Ref 13)

GROUP I: Statutorily accepted homeless individuals and households

Description

This group comprises the priority need categories specified in current legislation. They are predominantly couples with children,

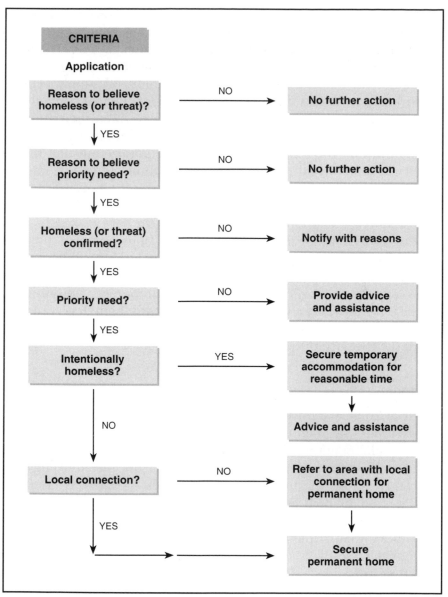

CRITERIA

Application

Reason to believe homeless (or threat)? — NO → No further action

↓ YES

Reason to believe priority need? — NO → No further action

↓ YES

Homeless (or threat) confirmed? — NO → Notify with reasons

↓ YES

Priority need? — NO → Provide advice and assistance

↓ YES

Intentionally homeless? — YES → Secure temporary accommodation for reasonable time

↓ NO

↓ → Advice and assistance

Local connection? — NO → Refer to area with local connection for permanent home

↓ YES

↓ → Secure permanent home

Fig 1.1 *The criteria used to establish that an applicant for housing is accepted as homeless and their effect on securing a permanent home.* (Source: *Housing the homeless: the local authority role.* Audit Commission, 1989) (Ref 13)

single parents, pregnant women or others who are deemed to be 'vulnerable'. They are frequently placed by local authorities in temporary accommodation such as bed and breakfast (B&B) hotels, hostels, short-life housing, private-sector housing ('private sector

leased') and 'homeless at home' schemes. Temporary accommodation is often used whilst their circumstances are being investigated
to see if they qualify under the law, as well as after they have formally
been accepted as homeless. The growing use of temporary accommodation is, at least in part, due to the reduced supply of local
authority permanent housing (see page 25). It may be argued that
people in Group I are not in fact homeless, since their housing
need has been officially accepted. This conclusion, however, fails to
recognise that their accommodation is temporary and that this in
itself can affect health status. A high proportion of these people are
not recorded as having been found permanent housing.[13] Such
households may 'disappear' from official statistics because, unable
to tolerate the temporary accommodation they are placed in, they
opt to try to fend for themselves again in a housing system that was
unable to provide for them in the first place. Others will 'reappear'
on official statistics after failing in such attempts.[13] Both households
who remain for prolonged periods in 'temporary' housing and
those who move in and out of the 'statutorily homeless' category
lack secure and health-maintaining living space, and this situation
underlies the health risks that they encounter.

Statistics

Official homelessness statistics are a useful source of information on
households* deemed to be in priority need and placed in temporary accommodation.[14] The quarterly records give numbers according to placements in 'B&B', 'hostels' and 'short-life housing etc'.
Table 1.1 shows the number of households accepted as homeless
and placed in B&B accommodation. Although there has been a
sharp decline in England in 1992, the number of such households
has more than tripled over the past decade. Two-thirds of local
authorities use B&B, and many, particularly in London, use hotels
in other boroughs.[8] Movement between hotels at short notice, and
at the request of placing authorities rather than homeless people
themselves, is not uncommon. Such inappropriate placement and
mobility lead to numerous problems concerning health status and
access to health, education and social services (Chapter 3). The use
of B&B has fallen in London since 1990 with more use being made
of privately leased accommodation.

---

*The unit used in official statistics is the 'household', which may consist of a
single person or a large family. The household figures should be multiplied by
2.8 to estimate the number of individuals.[21]

TABLE 1.1   **Households accepted as homeless by local authorities and placed in bed & breakfast hotels, 1980–1992**

Year	England (No.)	Wales (No.)	Scotland (No.)
1980	1,330	67	33
1981	1,520	63	178
1982	1,640	21	305
1983	2,700	17	279
1984	3,670	31	499
1985	5,360	20	335
1986	8,990	35	392
1987	10,370	45	213
1988	10,970	41	201
1989	11,480	173	317
1990	11,130	141	328
1991	12,120[a]	242[a]	458
1992	7,710[a]	248[a]	616

Sources: DOE, England; Welsh Office; Scottish Office.
Note: Figures for England and Wales show numbers in this accommodation at end of 4th quarter; Scotland figures are for end of 1st quarter.
[a]Excludes intentionally homeless.

Table 1.2 shows the number of officially accepted homeless households living in hostels for the years 1980–92. The figures show a sustained rise and largely reflect the supply of suitable hostel accommodation rather than need or demand. Table 1.3 shows the trend in the number of officially accepted homeless households placed in short-life and other types of temporary accommodation, including privately leased housing. The numbers have risen from 4,200 in England in 1982 to 44,490 in 1992. There were 8,574 Group I homeless households in B&B hotels in Great Britain in 1992.*

The current proposals for fundamental changes in the homelessness legislation will have profound effects on Group I homeless people (see Chapter 6).

---

*This is the number of households residing in B&B at a specific point during the year (end of 4th quarter in England and Wales, end of 1st quarter in Scotland). The total number of households placed in B&B during the year is not reflected in these figures.

TABLE 1.2 **Households accepted as homeless by local authorities and placed in hostels, 1980–1992**

Year	England (No.)	Wales[b] (No.)	Scotland (No.)
1980	3,380	147	33
1981	3,320	174	86
1982	3,500	113	97
1983	3,400	111	59
1984	3,990	109	73
1985	4,730	127	102
1986	4,610	148	210
1987	5,150	172	389
1988	6,240	233	362
1989	8,020	204	383
1990	9,010	310	579
1991	10,070[a]	354	1,363
1992	10,740[a]	326	1,384

Sources: DOE, England; Welsh Office; Scottish Office.
Note: England and Wales, 4th quarter; Scotland, 1st quarter.
[a]Excludes intentionally homeless.
[b]Local authority hostels only.

GROUP II: Rough sleepers, night shelter, direct-access hostel and B&B hotel single homeless people

Although clearly visible to the public, Group II homeless people are not recognised by the Government as homeless and are technically part of the unofficial, 'hidden' homeless population.

Description

The people described as Group II in this report live and sleep on the streets, or use night shelters, DHSS resettlement centres, common lodging houses or direct-access hostels, or they live in B&B hotels. Unlike Group I, those comprising Group II have not been accepted by a local authority as statutorily homeless. They may refer themselves to B&B, or be sent by a voluntary agency. Group II homeless

TABLE 1.3 **Households accepted as homeless by local authorities and placed in short-life housing etc, 1982–1992**

Year	England (No.)	Wales (No.)	Scotland (No.)
1982	4,200	334	254
1983	3,740	362	391
1984	4,640	354	351
1985	5,830	315	526
1986	7,190	310	782
1987	9,240	442	819
1988	12,890	380	947
1989	18,400	455	983
1990	25,030	560	1,216
1991	37,790[a]	618	1,334
1992	44,490[a]	458	1,435

Sources: DOE, England; Welsh Office; Scottish Office.
Note: England and Wales, 4th quarter; Scotland, 1st quarter.
[a]Excludes intentionally homeless.

people may move between hostels, night shelters and B&B hotels. Some intermittently or continuously sleep rough, although a 1991–2 survey has shown that the movement between rough sleeping and hostel or B&B living is not extensive.[15] Despite such survey information, many facts about Group II homelessness are unknown. Some people find a route out of homelessness by being deemed 'vulnerable' and thus accepted for housing by local authorities. Group II, the majority of whom are single white men, constitutes a relatively distinct population with characteristic patterns of health needs and problems.[7,8,15,16] Though women are found in this population they are much less numerous; a variety of reasons have been offered to explain this.[8,15,17,18]

Statistics

Rough sleepers

The 1991 census attempted to enumerate the people who were sleeping on the streets of Britain on census night. The numbers and

certain characteristics of this population are shown in Table 1.4.
They are predominantly white males, with few adolescents and few
pensioners.[19] Limited information is also available from other
sources, such as a survey carried out in London by a research team
on behalf of the Salvation Army. This included a direct count of
rough sleepers in sample areas.[20] They found 750 rough sleepers in
the 17 boroughs they studied and concluded that the number of
'visibly homeless' rough sleepers in all 33 London boroughs in April
1989 was 2,000. Another much quoted figure comes from the campaigning charity Shelter, which estimated that in 1992 there were

TABLE 1.4   **Socio-demographic characteristics of rough sleepers who were
enumerated by the 1991 census, Great Britain**

Characteristic	England (No.)	Wales (No.)	Scotland (No.)
Total numbers:	*2,650*	*32*	*145*
Gender			
Male	2,243	30	124
Female	407	2	21
Age group:			
0–15	0	2	1
16–17	35	0	1
18–29	1,013	13	26
30–44	842	9	54
45–59	657	5	52
60–64	55	1	5
65–74	37	0	5
75 and over	11	0	1
Economic activity:			
In employment	113	2	1
Unemployed	901	9	65
Economically inactive[a]	1,636	19	78
Ethnic group:			
Black	52	0	1
White	2,566	32	143
Indian, Pakistani and Bangladeshi	10	0	0
Chinese and other	18	0	0

Note: Subtotals do not always add to total because of missing data.
Source: Adapted from: *Communal establishments*, Census 1991. London: HMSO,
1993. (Ref 19)
[a]Economically inactive means not in gainful employment and not currently
seeking work.

2,000–3,000 rough sleepers in London and a further 3,000 in other parts of Britain.[21] A recently published study described single homeless people who were not officially accepted as homeless by local authorities. Three groups were surveyed: those living in hostels or B&B hotels, and two groups of rough sleepers—those attending day centres and those using soup-runs.[15] Table 1.5 shows certain socio-demographic features of these three groups. Again they comprise largely a white male population of middle years. A large proportion of them have no educational qualifications, and many have

TABLE 1.5 **Selected socio-demographic characteristics and experience of institutional living of Group II homeless people**

	Hostel and B&B (%)	Day centre (%)	Soup run (%)
Male	77	93	87
Female	23	7	13
Age group:			
16–17	5	2	3
18–24	25	13	16
25–44	36	47	46
45–59	18	28	28
60+	14	10	7
White	73	96	99
Black	16	1	0
Indian, Pakistani or Bangladeshi	2	1	0
Other ethnic group	8	1	1
Whether in paid work in previous week	10	7	6
Median income in previous week (£)	39	39	37
Possess no educational qualifications	53	62	NA
Whether ever stayed:			
– in a children's home	15	24	24
– in prison or remand centre	25	49	46
– in general hospital for over 3 months	10	22	20
– in psychiatric hospital/unit	12	20	17
(*Base numbers*)	*1,267*	*345*	*152*

Source: Adapted from *Single homeless people.* London: HMSO, 1993. (Ref 15)
NA = Not available.

spent time in residential institutions such as children's homes, prisons and general or psychiatric hospitals.

It is technically difficult to estimate the number of rough sleepers.[22,23] Many such people understandably conceal their resting sites to reduce the risk of violence. Their choice of site may vary according to the weather and they may change sites rapidly and unpredictably. Many see enumeration as an intrusion and actively avoid it. Their numbers fall in the short term when temporary hostel places are provided. For reasons such as these, the 1991 census data are thought to underestimate considerably the number of rough sleepers. For example, the census recorded no rough sleepers in Birmingham, while researchers six months later identified 60.[22] Similar differences were observed in Oxford and emphasise the need for better enumeration techniques.[22,23]

Hostel dwellers

A *hostel* may be one of a large variety of relatively distinct types of temporary accommodation.[24] Some hostels still conform to the stereotype of a large institution, providing very short-stay (one night) accommodation in dormitory type settings. These are generally open to all-comers (direct access), and many offer very poor living conditions and little or no privacy. Some do not guarantee accommodation for more than a single night and are better called 'night shelters'. The outmoded term 'common lodging house' denotes an intermediate category. Yet another descriptive term derives from the former Department of Health and Social Security (DHSS) which set up and ran a number of large hostels known as DHSS Resettlement Units. Many commentators, including the DHSS, have criticised these facilities and as a result, a programme of closure is now under way. Although 22 DHSS resettlement units remained in 1992, all are due to be closed. The intention is to provide smaller hostels offering a variety of social and, less frequently, health care services. Such hostels may be funded by local authorities, the Housing Corporation,* the voluntary sector or any combination of these. Many plan to set specific criteria for admission, and therefore will not provide direct access. Most of them offer a more domiciliary style of accommodation.[24] Although this trend is generally welcome, there remains concern that direct-access hostel places are being closed without adequate replacement.

---

*This is the organisation funded by central government which registers and disperses funding to registered housing associations and, since 1988, has been given additional powers to 'approve' landlords in the social-rented sector.

The wide range of facilities labelled 'hostel' makes it difficult to determine accurately the number of direct-access hostel dwellers who are not accepted as statutorily homeless. The figure can perhaps be estimated from the difference between the total number of available bed-spaces (22,383 in London and 37,759 in the rest of England at the end of 1991)[25] and the number of persons statutorily accepted as homeless. This gives the number of Group II *unofficial* homeless people in hostels in England in 1991, at the end of the 4th quarter, as around 50,000.

The 1991 census provided information on the number and socio-demographic characteristics of people residing in 'hostels and

TABLE 1.6 **Numbers and socio-demographic characteristics of persons residing in hostels and common lodging houses enumerated by the 1991 census, Great Britain**

	England (No.)	Wales (No.)	Scotland (No.)
Total numbers:	*16,346*	*594*	*2,477*
Males	11,189	398	2,009
Females	5,157	196	468
Age group:			
0–15	1,591	100	92
16–17	629	18	60
18–29	5,395	163	405
30–44	3,246	116	427
45–PA	3,602	137	951
PA and over	1,883	60	542
In employment	2,776	54	197
Unemployed	5,320	133	849
Economically inactive[a]	6,659	307	1,339
White	13,617	559	2,451
Black	1,563	11	11
Indian, Pakistani and Bangladeshi	496	10	7
Chinese and other	670	14	8

Source: Adapted from: *Communal establishments*, Census 1991. London: HMSO, 1993. (Ref 19)
PA = Pensionable age.
[a]Economically inactive means not in gainful employment and not currently seeking work.

common lodging houses' on census night (Table 1.6). The data are essentially similar to those for rough sleepers. It is not possible to analyse this figure into those placed by local authorities, those self-referred and those residing in a hostel for reasons other than housing need. It refers to direct-access hostel and common lodging house users and excludes housing association hostels, whereas the estimate above includes all hostel types (eg bail hostels). A working party of the Single Homeless in London (SHIL) which surveyed London hostels used mainly by single homeless people in June 1988 estimated that there were 11,500 homeless people in such London hostels. However in a study conducted one year later, using different methods, the number of single homeless people in London hostels was estimated at 18,000.[20]

Bed and breakfast dwellers

A final component of Group II homeless people are those not accepted as statutorily homeless and who come to live in B&B hotels through referring themselves or after being referred by an agency. The size of this group is unknown, though in the representative sampling method adopted by Anderson *et al* they made up 25% of the sample.[15] This study highlighted the changing socio-demographic characteristics of Group II homeless people and reported a growing proportion of those aged under 21 years, and of females. Other studies have also revealed the increasing problem of youth homelessness.[7,8,16,21]

Explanations offered for the increase in homelessness among young people include the difficulties faced by unskilled workers in an increasingly competitive labour market.[8] It has been suggested that the abolition of the right of persons aged 16 and 17 years to non-discretionary income support, and the reduced amount paid to those aged 18–24, has increased the vulnerability of young people to homelessness.[8,21,26] Many children and youths may also become homeless because, in addition to these factors, they are attempting to escape an abusing family or an inadequate child care placement.[26,27] In addition, some young people are ill-equipped or may be unwilling to accept the obligations and responsibilities of adult society. The combination of factors for each individual is complex, but the shortage of economic resources and employment opportunities faced by young people should be accorded as much weight as explanations based upon personal characteristics.

A further particularly vulnerable group among Group II homeless people are those suffering from a serious mental illness (see Chapter 5).

GROUP III: Other groups in housing need

Description

This group comprises all those with significant housing need who are not Group I homeless and do not fall into Group II. Some, such as single parents about to be made homeless by relatives, are eligible under the 1985 Housing Act for official recognition, but the majority are not. People in this group are in insecure accommodation (see Box 2). The majority of them are *concealed* households and a proportion of them are *potential* households. The term 'concealed household' refers to the situation where two or more households share accommodation but are counted as a single household in the census. The term 'potential household' refers to a situation where the concealed household or members of a household wish to live separately. As might be expected, single-person potential households are the largest group who fail to fulfil the legal criteria for homelessness.[7,8,28] The second largest group of potential households comprise couples without dependent children. Such people may, of course, seek public-sector rehousing by other means, such as joining a local authority housing list.

Statistics

Estimating the size of the Group III hidden homeless is beset with problems and there are no reliable official UK estimates. This gap in our knowledge is due largely to the absence of a current systematic survey of housing need. The last official study was the National Dwelling and Housing Survey, conducted in England and Wales in the 1970s and published in 1979.[29] Recently, however, estimates of the current number of potential households in England obtained in a survey of sharers has become available (Box 4).[30]

CAUSES OF HOMELESSNESS

For many years in the UK both health and housing policy were key central components of the welfare state. However, since the 1980s there has been continuing debate about the proper role of the state in providing access to services or resources such as health care, housing, education and income,[31-34] and there have been significant changes in the role the state seeks to play in providing housing through local authorities and housing associations. Essentially, central government has shifted support from local government to

BOX 4

Concealed and potential households: survey of sharers, England 1990

This survey defined three groups of sharers:

Group A   Households were classified as *living in non self-contained accommodation* if they shared a kitchen, bathroom or toilet with another household, or if they shared circulation space with other households. Such households form about 1.5–2% of the population.

Group B   A *concealed family* was defined as a unit of two or more persons living in a larger household headed by someone who was not a member of the concealed family unit. A concealed family could consist of a married or cohabiting couple with or without children, or a lone parent and child(ren).

Group C   The survey covered three groups of *concealed adults*: unmarried (ie not currently married) people aged 18 or over living with parents; unmarried people aged 16 or over living with other relatives; and unmarried people aged 16 or over living with non-relatives.

		Group A	**Group B**	**Group C**
N	Numbers) (000s)	278–371	260	3600[a] 500[b] 700[c]
P	Percentage who would strongly prefer self-contained accommodation[d]			11[a] 4[b]
		40	28	9[c]
$N \times P$	Numbers (000s) of potential households	111–148	73	396[a] 20[b] 63[c]

[a]Unmarried people living with parents.
[b]Unmarried people not living with parents but related to household head.
[c]Unmarried people not living with parents and not related to the household head.
[d]Whether or not they could afford this.

Source: *Shared accommodation in England, 1990.* London: OPCS, 1992. (Ref 30)

housing associations which are now viewed as the main providers of rented accommodation for people who are unable or unwilling to become home-owners.[31] The principal agent of this policy is the Housing Corporation which registers housing associations, approves new building schemes and dispenses government grants.

The causes of homelessness are complex and multiple. Detailed analyses are given elsewhere.[8,16,18] Only a brief review of the evidence is presented here, taking account particularly of the balance between housing need and housing supply. Social and economic factors such as family structure and employment can be shown to be associated with homelessness, but it is difficult to assign causation in respect of individuals. Ill health may increase the risk of homelessness (Chapter 2). Official statistics record reasons for homelessness amongst households accepted by local authorities as having priority need, but these are widely regarded as simple administrative categories which, at best, reflect the final problem in a causal chain leading to homelessness.[8,17,18] The major reason recorded in the official statistics is 'homelessness because friends and relatives are no longer willing to accommodate'. However, such events are reasons for homelessness only within the context of particular social and economic frameworks. Thus, low levels of income do not inevitably and necessarily lead to homelessness, especially if social policy accords priority to affordable housing.[8,15,18]

Most analyses of the causes of homelessness in the UK focus on the mismatch between the level of housing need in the population and the supply and accessibility of housing in three sectors: the public sector (local authority and housing association rented sectors, also termed the social-rented sector), the private-rented sector, and the home-ownership sector.

Housing need

Even though there is no agreement regarding the point on the spectrum where housing need (see Box 2) becomes 'real' or 'legitimate', traditional indicators such as the official homelessness statistics (Table 1.7) and other indicators such as local authority housing waiting list numbers and house repossession figures show that the trend level of need is increasing.[28] The reductions in official homelessness in 1992 and 1993 are thought to reflect a tightening of acceptances by local authorities owing to the severe shortage of permanent housing available to them.

Homelessness is not only a London problem. Both the absolute numbers and the annual rate of increase are rising faster outside

TABLE 1.7   **Statutorily accepted homeless households, Great Britain**

Year	England (No.)	Wales (No.)	Scotland (No.)	Great Britain (Total No.)
1978	53,110	3,204	6,699	63,013
1979	57,200	4,676	8,356	70,232
1980	62,920	5,446	8,105	76,471
1981	70,010	5,462	8,149	83,621
1982	74,800	5,611	9,303	89,714
1983	78,240	5,008	8,919	92,167
1984	83,550	4,999	9,727	98,276
1985	93,980	5,371	12,406	111,757
1986	103,560	5,965	13,349	122,874
1987	112,440	5,683	12,637	130,760
1988	117,500	6,818	12,601	136,919
1989	126,680	7,794	14,391	148,865
1990	145,800	8,670	15,056	169,526
1991	145,140[a]	9,813	17,800	177,283
1992	142,000[a]	10,311	17,655	169,966
1993	134,190[a]	10,879	NA	NA

Sources: DOE, England; Scottish Office; Welsh Office.
Note: Scottish figures are published by financial year and refer to households
accepted as priority homeless. The figures are not therefore directly comparable.
[a]Excludes intentionally homeless not permanently rehoused.
NA = Not available.

London.[35] Nor is it solely an urban issue as rural homelessness is a
large and growing problem.[36] For our present purpose, the availability of accommodation providing a safe, continuing and quality
environment is seen as a prerequisite for health.[7] Estimating housing need, in terms of the number of homes required in the UK to
further these health objectives, yields a figure far in excess of
current and projected levels of private and public sector output.
If hidden homelessness is included as a legitimate category of
homelessness the numbers in need increase dramatically. In particular, if potential households consisting of single parents and couples,

and the backlog of housing replacements (required because of unfit housing conditions) are included, the estimated number of *additional* homes required in England alone is 60,000 per year over the period 1991–2001.[37] The estimate already given of the number of current potential households in England is based on the results of the survey of sharers (Box 4). An estimate in 1989 for England and Wales led to the figure of between 100,000 and 1.2 million potential households, with cogent arguments favouring the higher end of this range.[28] This estimate, unlike those used in census-derived projections of housing need, included single-person potential households, which raises significantly the need for additional housing.[37]

Changes in family composition are key factors in the determination of future needs for housing.[37] Birth, marriage and divorce all have an influence on the demand and need for housing. There is, for example, a pronounced trend in the UK towards one-person households; they made up 25% of all households in 1986 and are expected to represent 31% by 2001.[28] However, simply using population projections of census-type households is not an adequate method of calculating housing need. It does not adjust the projected figure for the likely growth in potential households, and it does not take into account the need to replace unfit housing. It also disregards the geographical mismatch between need and supply of housing.[37] Box 5 shows a recent attempt to take these factors into account to arrive at a 'social housing' system for England that meets housing need in the year 2001.* The annual output of social-rented housing in England between 1991 and 2001 that is required to meet current and projected needs lies between 53,000 and 141,000. If single-person potential households are included, this rises to between 63,000 and 151,000 with a likely central estimate of 110,000.[37] Even with favourable current assumptions about the output of social-rented housing, there will be a shortfall of about 70,000 homes per year.[37]

Supply and accessibility of housing

The supply of housing has to be considered in relation to its accessibility to those in need. A supply that is large but economically, geographically or organisationally inaccessible makes no contribution to the reduction of need.

---

*Social housing comprises the local authority and housing association rented sectors.

BOX 5

+---+

**Estimation model* to produce an annual output of social
housing which meets specified needs by 2001, England**

	No. per annum
Backlog	10,000
Vacancy rates at 4%	25,000
Concealed households	26,000
Mismatch	10,000
Overlap between backlog and concealed	5,000
Gross stock minus census households ('mechanistic surplus')	26,500
Total (additional social provision required)	62,500
Assumed social output on current trends	40,000
Total social requirement	*102,500*

*Kleinmann and Whitehead, gross-flow model.

+---+

Source: *A review of housing needs assessment.* London: Housing Corporation, 1992.
(Ref 37)

There are four sectors of housing provision:

> Home-ownership
> Privately rented housing
> Local authority housing
> Housing association rented housing } social rented sector

Home-ownership is seen by many politicians, policy makers and the general public in the UK as the 'normal' tenure type.[8] However, comparison with other countries shows that a high level of home-ownership is not universal.[38] In the UK, home-ownership is heavily subsidised (around £6 billion in 1992) by central government via mortgage interest relief which has been criticised as inequitable, inefficient and inflationary.[18,39] The reconvened Inquiry into British Housing, under the chairmanship of HRH The Duke of Edinburgh, recommended phasing out this subsidy.[40] The reduction in mortgage interest relief in the 1993 Budget is a move in this direction.

Most commentators believe that the level of UK home-ownership has reached an economically feasible ceiling with around 68% of households now owning their homes outright or via a mortgage.[18,31]

Since 1981 the accessibility of home-ownership has been significantly increased for local authority tenants, who have been able to purchase their homes at up to 70% discounts via the 'right to buy' policy. Research has shown that people who purchase through this scheme are, in general, those who are in employment and have earnings at the top end of the income distribution of local authority tenants.[31] The right to buy policy has undoubtedly opened up home-ownership to thousands of households, but it has also transferred housing from relatively accessible local authority renting to the less accessible home-ownership sector.[7,18,31,41] An unforeseen consequence of the right to buy policy has been a process of *residualisation* of the remaining local authority sector. This means that properties in poorer condition, in unattractive sites, are left in local authority ownership whilst the more desirable and better maintained properties have been bought.[31,41] Residualisation is a term also applied to remaining local authority tenants, both those who did not buy and those newly entering this tenure. An increasing proportion of local authority tenants are socio-economically disadvantaged compared with home-owners. This situation has been described as *polarisation*[41] (Table 1.8).

Home-ownership remains economically inaccessible to a sizeable proportion of the UK population.[7,18,31,42] Despite recent falls in the price of houses, this situation is not set to change in the future. Many commentators have concluded that a more equitable housing finance system is needed, with a reduction in the subsidy enjoyed by home-owners accompanied by a mortgage benefit payment for home-owners in financial difficulty.[43]

Privately rented housing was the norm around the turn of the century. Since then the sector has declined substantially and now accounts for only 7% of all UK households. The privately rented sector has traditionally been the main source of affordable housing for low-income tenants who either actively choose it or use it as a 'tenure of last resort'.[7,8,31] Nowadays there are two main groups using this tenure: young relatively affluent people intending to move into home-ownership, and low-income people unable to access any other tenure. Affordability of rents remains a problem.[8,21,31] Means-tested housing benefit results, in many cases, in a benefit 'poverty trap' (which applies also to the social-rented sector) because a recipient who gets a job will suffer a steep

TABLE 1.8 **Residualisation effects: heads of households renting from a local authority, Great Britain, 1981, 1987, 1989**

Characteristic	1981 (%)	1987 (%)	1989 (%)
Gross Weekly Median Income as a % of median for all heads of households in each economic activity category:			
Economically active	82	63	59
Economically inactive[a]	102	86	82
Households economically inactive[a]	42	57	60
Household heads aged 65 or over	31	39	39
Households in lower half of income distribution	—	81	81
Households with 2 or more bedrooms above standard (occupancy indicator):			
Owned with mortgage	25	27	31
Local authority rented	13	14	13

Source: Adapted from: *General Household Survey 1989.* London: HMSO, 1991.
[a]Economically inactive means not in gainful employment and not currently seeking work.

reduction in benefit in relation to earnings.

In an attempt to increase the availability of privately rented housing, the 1988 Housing Act introduced significant changes which deregulated private renting. The intention was to make renting more attractive to potential landlords.[31] The principal elements of the deregulation were the abolition of security of tenure, which was replaced by assured tenancy contracts, and the scrapping of the 'fair rents' system, replacing it with 'market rents'. However, the central problem with the private-rented sector remains the low return on investment available to landlords.[28,31] In essence, commercially viable rents are too high for low-income families.[26,27,35] It has been estimated that in England alone there are 764,000 empty private properties that could be rented. Many of these could be let at once, while others require renovation. It is estimated that the cost of keeping properties empty (maintenance, deterioration, insurance and security) is £30–100 million per 10,000 homes.[44] A revival of this sector could play a major part in reducing homelessness, but this requires policies to make private renting attractive to landlords and affordable to tenants.

Local authority housing (council housing) enjoyed an uncontroversial position for a time after World War II, when it was seen by all parties as a solution to 'general housing needs'. Since the 1950s this consensus has broken down.[31] Today local authorities are enjoined by central government to be 'enablers' of housing choice rather than landlords or managers of housing.[31] Consequently the supply of local authority housing has declined significantly (Fig 1.2), owing to the generally unfavourable financial incentives for new building schemes.[31,42]

The sale of council houses with the associated fall in the quantity and quality of local authority housing has led to growing social, economic and health disparities between local authority tenants and home-owners.[18,31,41] The increased demand for and reduced supply

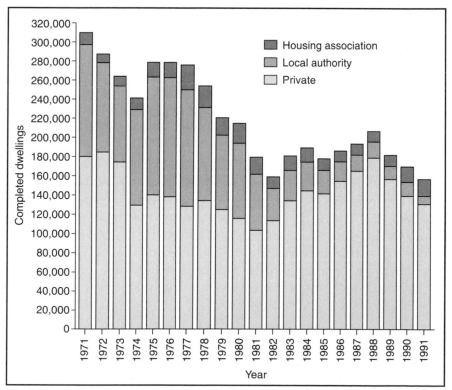

Fig 1.2 *Total number of completed dwellings in England and Wales 1971–1991, by sector.*

of local authority housing means that waiting lists have grown. Consequently applicants not deemed to be in priority need are unlikely to be allocated a council house within a reasonable time.[45,46] Non-priority applicants and others sometimes blame homeless households for 'jumping the queue'. This argument underpins the proposed fundamental changes in the homelessness legislation.[47] Such a view, however, represents a misunderstanding of the role of local authorities in a severely reduced social rented sector,[13] and ignores the need for a housing policy which safeguards and promotes health (see Chapter 6).

Housing association rented housing is now promoted as the primary source of social housing in the UK. At present about 3% of UK households are accommodated in this sector. This proportion will grow with increasing implementation of the 1988 Housing Act which allows the transfer of ownership and management of local authority housing stock to housing associations. Traditionally this sector provided for groups with special needs, such as elderly people, rather than statutorily accepted homeless households. Local authorities are now, however, attempting to meet their responsibilities for homeless people through rights that allow them to nominate about 50% of new tenancies in the housing association sector.

The grant element in the subsidy from the Housing Corporation to housing associations has fallen from 95% to 62%, with an intention to reduce it in future to 55%. This fall in grant has led to large increases in rental charges because there are no policy sanctions to control rents, which therefore rise to the level allowed by housing benefit regulations. This tenure has thus become less affordable and accessible to low-income households caught in a benefit poverty trap.[18,31] Consequently, people who are low-paid but do not qualify for housing benefit have an incentive to avoid this tenure. New entrants are thus characterised by increasingly high levels of unemployment, and this increases social marginalisation. The appropriateness of segregating deprived households in this way is hard to justify and, at the very least, raises questions about their acceptance and integration in the community.[48]

CONCLUSIONS

The housing system in the UK at present appears to be unable to ensure the availability of housing on the basis of need. Home-ownership remains impossible for a significant section of the population, and there has been a continuous decline in both the accessibility and availability of local authority and private sector rented housing. Housing associations remain minor providers of housing, and even if they achieve an annual output of 40,000 new lettings this will still fall short of need.[28,36,37,45] There is a supply and affordability crisis in UK housing which, as subsequent chapters will show, has important consequences for health.

RECOMMENDATION 1

The statistics collected on homelessness should be expanded to include rough sleepers and direct-access hostel dwellers (Group II homeless) and such people should be *officially* recognised as homeless.

References to Chapter 1 appear on page 125.

2 Health and housing opportunities

SUMMARY

The relationships between health and access to housing are complex, but there is evidence that health status and disability can adversely affect housing opportunities:

- Ill and disabled people are more likely than others to be unemployed or in low-paid jobs.

- Income is necessary to obtain adequate housing in the home-ownership and private-rented sectors.

- The social-rented sector, which provides housing based on need rather than ability to pay, has decreased in size, making access more difficult.

- The homelessness legislation and medical priority for rehousing (MPR) systems might, in theory, ensure that ill health and disability do not reduce access to housing. However, in practice, these systems cannot guarantee that health needs are addressed in the allocation of social housing.

- Ill health can therefore limit housing opportunities.

INTRODUCTION

Until 1951 central government responsibility for housing was placed within the Ministry of Health. This reflected the view long-held by politicians and society that housing conditions were closely connected with health status, and indeed the improvements in housing during the 19th century were brought about through laws dealing with public health.[1]

Today, even within the continuing debate on the proper role of Government in the provision of resources such as housing, there remains broad support for the continuation of policies that serve as a 'safety net' for those who are generally considered to be unable to provide for themselves. Some groups are, under the 1985 Housing Act, accorded legal rights to permanent housing ('priority home-lessness groups'), whilst others are accorded statutory rights to housing only if they are deemed 'vulnerable'. The designation of a category of vulnerable people implies a *prima facie* acceptance of the following or a closely similar argument:

  i People who suffer from a chronic illness or disability that curtails their functioning, or from a recurrent illness that interferes with their working capacity, will experience certain disadvantages in the labour market.

 ii Employment and income are pivotal factors in determining success in the housing market.

   It therefore follows that:

iii Ill health can exert an adverse influence on housing opportunities.

   In this chapter we argue that ill health reduces housing opportunities. To establish this we will look in turn at the relationships between housing and employment, employment and health, and housing and health. The overall analysis rests on the view that there is a 'health selection effect' relating to housing, as set out in a UK context by Smith.[1] She argues that ill health operates to reduce housing opportunities, and that the mechanisms which might redress this, such as the 'medical priority for rehousing' (MPR) system, are in practice inadequate to do so.

HOUSING OPPORTUNITIES, EMPLOYMENT AND HEALTH

Housing and employment

Within the UK housing system it is apparent that ability to pay dictates access to two sectors: home-ownership and private renting. Employment is the crucial determinant in house buying and in being able to sustain this tenure.[2-5] Of those people officially accepted as homeless, 10–12% have become so because of their inability to service a mortgage.[6] Moreover, the affordability of home-ownership increasingly rests on the availability of two incomes, and thus interruption of employment, even for one member of a couple, may be a determining factor in mortgage arrears.[4,5,7] In the privately rented sector, despite the existence and expansion of

TABLE 2.1   **Socio-economic group of household heads by tenure type, Great Britain 1989**

	Owner occupied		Rented		
	Owned outright (%)	With mortgage (%)	Local authority (%)	Housing assoc. (%)	Private (%)
Economically active:					
Professional	3	9	0	0	5
Employers and managers	9	26	1	1	10
Intermediate non-manual	4	12	2	3	9
Junior non-manual	3	7	4	7	8
Skilled-manual and non-professional	12	30	17	16	15
Skilled-manual and personal service	3	8	11	9	8
Unskilled manual	2	2	4	3	3
Economically inactive[a]	65	7	59	61	45
Total	*100*	*100*	*100*	*100*	*100*

Source: Adapted from: Table 8.60 of the *General Household Survey 1989.* London: HMSO, 1991.
Note: Figures may not add to 100 because of rounding.
[a]Economically inactive means not in gainful employment and not currently seeking work.

housing benefit payments, employment still remains a crucial factor in determining access, sustainability and quality of housing.[2–4]

   The remaining sectors form the *social-rented sector,* in which the influence of employment on accessibility and affordability becomes less distinct. This sector is now the principal focus of housing policy in the welfare state, within which the allocation of housing is based on need rather than on ability to pay. It is therefore not surprising that the socio-economic (Table 2.1) and employment characteristics (Table 2.2) of those in the various sectors differ systematically. However, employment status remains important even for people who do gain access to social-rented housing. They are more likely to

TABLE 2.2   **Employment status of new heads of households entering tenures in the previous year, 1984**

	Owner occupied (%)	Local authority rented (%)	Private rented (%)	Housing association rented (%)
Employed	90	34	62	74
Unemployed	3	27	16	25
Retired	2	7	2	—
Other economically inactive[a]	5	32	20	1
Bases	*220,000*	*150,000*	*190,000*	*20,000*

Source: Adapted from: *Housing trailers to the 1984 labour force survey.*
London: HMSO, 1988. (Ref 8)
[a]Economically inactive means not in gainful employment and not currently seeking work.

be unemployed during economic downturns than those in owner occupation. This risk persists even when the occupational distributions between tenures and regional patterns of employment are taken into account.[8] Moreover, despite the persistence of the welfare state principle of need rather than ability to pay, rents in the social-rented sector are rising in real terms, and rent arrears are increasing,[3,9,10] so that affordability cannot be taken for granted. Indeed, rent arrears may disqualify households from the statutory homelessness procedures, because their homelessness is deemed 'intentional'. There are wide variations in the practices of local authorities: 9% of London authorities compared with 51% of non-metropolitan authorities said they would not accept rent arrears cases. Overall, 45% of local authorities in England and Wales do not accept such cases as eligible for rehousing under the homelessness legislation.[11]

The importance of employment in determining accessibility and affordability of housing is emphasised by the high rates of unemployment among people accepted by local authorities as homeless.[2,3,11]

Employment and health

The relationships between health and employment are complex. Even within the same occupational category there appear to be systematic differences in disease risk between different grades which cannot be accounted for solely by lifestyle differences.[12] In the UK, social class is based on occupation, and systematic associations between social class and both morbidity and mortality are well documented.[12,13] The possible explanations for this persistent association were thoroughly discussed by a working group on inequalities in health,[12] which concluded that, although cultural and genetic factors contribute, material factors are more important.

Employment status, labour market position and income are central determinants of the level of material resources available to an individual or household.[12-16] Unemployment has been found to increase risks of both morbidity and mortality.[12,15-19] During periods of economic restructuring, the impact of higher rates of unemployment falls disproportionately on the lower social classes, who are likely to have limited educational achievements, less transferable skills and to be less geographically mobile. Thus, employment opportunity is related to social class.[13,15]

Housing and health

The relationship between health status and housing opportunities involves a chain of reasoning which specifies, in its linking arguments, relationships that are not all-or-nothing but are based on probabilities. Housing opportunities, housing conditions, occupational social class, risk of unemployment and health risks are closely linked together in a web of reciprocal relationships. Within this web, one set of relationships is directly relevant to the existence of the health selection effect on housing opportunities (Fig 2.1). These *housing pathways* show how social and economic factors can interact with health status to increase the chances of living in poor quality housing or of becoming homeless. Further consideration must, however, be given to the social-rented sector, where allocation should be related to need rather than ability to pay. The allocation systems concerned are the homelessness legislation based on the 1985 Housing Act, and the 'medical priority for rehousing' (MPR) system (see Fig 2.1).

HOMELESSNESS LEGISLATION BASED ON THE 1985 (1977) HOUSING ACT

Current homelessness legislation recognises that certain groups of people have a statutory right to permanent housing (see

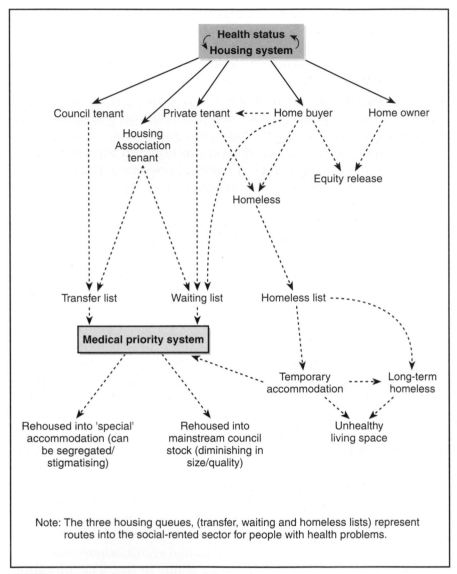

Fig 2.1 *Housing paths for people with health problems.* (From Smith SJ, Knill-Jones R, McGuckin A (eds). *Housing for health.* London: Longman. *(Ref 22)*

Chapter 1). People with a mental illness, mental handicap or a physical disability qualify for priority group status as 'vulnerable', and the law also allows those 'vulnerable by other special reason.'

The law concerning vulnerability has been substantially elaborated by case-law decisions. For example the meaning of 'vulnerability' was:

'. . . being less able to fend for oneself so that injury or detriment will result where a less vulnerable person will be able to cope without harmful effects.' This was further qualified as follows: '. . . the vulnerability should be relevant to the housing situation of the applicant'. (Quoted in Ref 3, pages 10 and 11)

In an analysis of case-law decisions it has been shown that ill health can be included as constituting vulnerability.[20] Consequently it may be reasoned that the present law, as it stands, has recognised the welfare 'safety net' function of housing with regard to ill health. The statutory system should ensure that no one is handicapped in securing adequate housing because of a labour market disadvantage related to health.

The emerging picture, however, suggests that there is a 'health selective effect' which results in people with ill health being not only less likely to receive housing that meets their needs but also at increased risk of homelessness.[1,21,22] The most direct evidence for a health selective effect comes from the health profile of homeless people. Chapters 3–5 of this report deal with this in detail and reveal that homeless people have a high prevalence of many types of disease.[1,3,21,22] This indicates that the present welfare 'safety net' approach to housing is not working adequately.[1,21,22] The explanations for this failure are multifaceted. Variations in acceptance policy between local authorities are increasingly recognised;[4,11] some authorities accept as homeless only 20% of all applicants, while others accept 80%.[23] Although no direct information is available about variations in practice related to vulnerability and health status, it is reasonable to suggest it is significant. Whereas 22% of all council waiting list applicants report a medical reason for seeking council housing, only 5% believe this reason has been accepted.[24] There are differences between local authority policies and also in the readiness of doctors to ascribe 'vulnerability' status.[1,21,22]

MEDICAL PRIORITY FOR REHOUSING

The allocation of housing on the basis of medical priority (see Fig 2.1) provides an alternative route to social-rented housing for people who are ill or disabled but not deemed to be in priority need.

The 'medical priority for rehousing' system is operated by local authorities and is meant to match housing to identified medical need.[1,21,22] People may place themselves on a local authority waiting list *de novo* or on a transfer list (if already in local authority accommodation) and ask for priority consideration because of medical need. However, there is accumulating evidence that there is considerable variation in the operation of this system and the effectiveness and efficiency of its implementation.[1,21,22,25] At present it does not provide an adequate counterweight to the disadvantages conferred by ill health.[25]

The inadequacies of the statutory homelessness procedures and the MPR system in responding to health needs are compounded by changes in the social-rented sector, which has decreased in size, desirability and accessibility.[25,26] The smaller social-rented stock means there is less scope for transfer to appropriate health-promoting housing via the MPR system, and this situation has major implications for the policy of community care (Box 6). Many factors[2,22,26,27] severely restrict the existing welfare 'safety net' systems which sought to ensure that disease and ill health would not discriminate against the achievement of health-promoting housing or, indeed, housing itself. The authors of the research summarised in Box 6 introduce their findings by stating:

> 'Better health, easier access to care and an enhanced quality of life are experienced by most people rehoused on medical grounds, a survey of 800 housing applicants in three urban authorities reveals. But according to interviews with housing providers, the effectiveness of this service is compromised by excess demand over supply. Case study evidence from nine local authorities suggests that better use of limited public resources might be made by linking medical rehousing to the aims of community care.'

Suggestions for this linkage are discussed in Chapter 6.

This discussion has focused on the inadequacies of existing systems in ensuring the implementation of the welfare ideal of accessible housing for people in poor health. It should be emphasised that the restricted supply of social-rented housing[3] results in the widespread use of temporary accommodation such as B&B hotels, short-life housing and hostels by people with health problems. Such accommodation cannot be considered suitable and does not represent adequate integration of housing needs with community care policies[22,28] (see Chapters 3–5).

BOX 6

**Medical Prioritisation for Rehousing (MPR) systems —
findings from recent research in England**

---

1   Health and mobility needs secure high priority in housing queues
    and medical priority rehousing has the following benefits:
    • Two-thirds of those rehoused attained homes which are in
      better overall repair, less likely to be damp or infested, easier to
      heat and less crowded than their previous dwellings.
    • Over 60% of those rehoused experienced health improve-
      ments; 70% are now happy and contented most or all of the
      time, compared with 15% of other movers.
    • Medical priority rehousing can reduce demand for local health
      services while improving access to care for those who still
      require it.

2   Despite these benefits only a minority of applicants secure
    priority rehousing. Most local authorities report recent increases
    in demand for medical rehousing yet, having sold up to 40% of
    their stock, find themselves with excess demand which is not
    accommodated by housing associations.

3   Those denied medical priority often experience their illness as
    acutely as those awarded it and two-thirds of non-movers believe
    their health has suffered.

4   Nearly half those denied a priority grading do not know why.
    Overall, 40% of applicants are dissatisfied with the service and say
    outcomes are unfair.

5   The stringent rationing of medical and mobility priority is
    causing frustration among health advisers, distress to house-
    holders and difficulties for sick or disabled homeless people and
    barriers to the integration of rehousing with community care
    strategies.

Source: Smith SJ *et al. Housing provision for people with health problems and mobility
difficulties.* York: Joseph Rowntree Foundation, 1993. (Ref 25)

RECOMMENDATION 2

The Government, local authorities, the Housing Corporation and the NHS should together undertake a wide-ranging
review of housing and community care policies, addressing
the opportunities for integration and the barriers to
progress. The aim should be to develop a co-ordinated

action plan that identifies and provides the organisational, management and resource requirements to allow the implementation and evaluation of a coherent joint policy.

RECOMMENDATION 3

Within the recommended joint policy, the current medical prioritisation procedures should be reviewed and integrated with community care and housing need assessment procedures. The conferment of priority need status should not prevent the assessment of housing need in relation to health need.

References to Chapter 2 appear on page 127.

3 Health problems of homeless families

SUMMARY

- The number of people who are *officially* homeless, mainly families with children and pregnant women, has risen dramatically over the past few years although the use of bed and breakfast accommodation has recently declined.

- The socio-demographic characteristics of the official homeless population differ markedly from those of rough sleepers and hostel dwellers.

- There is evidence of increased mental, physical and obstetric ill health compared with housed populations, and there are many clinical reports of increased ill health and behavioural problems, especially among the children.

- There are data showing a high rate of utilisation of both hospital and community services.

- There are particular problems for homeless families in gaining access to primary care.

- The social and financial disadvantages of homeless families make healthy lifestyles unattainable in most instances.

'I've always had a bad chest because I've got a weak heart, but my chest has got a lot worse, I cough a lot. My husband coughs a lot. We've got wheezy chests and my baby's got a wheezy chest, we've all been affected in that way. The mould I suppose because you get a lot of—it smells. And I've had a lot of stress as well just because of the state of the place, it just gets you down.'

'I was pregnant, I couldn't stay in bed and breakfast, because I wasn't eating properly, because I was getting very ill living off fish and chips all the time.'

'I go to the cafe down the road, but they only does chips and things like that, which is not a very good diet for the baby, like.'

'Well when you've got to wash, cook, clean, bloody live, sleep, argue in one room — you can't do it.'[22]

INTRODUCTION

This chapter presents evidence on the health effects of living in temporary accommodation, principally in bed and breakfast (B&B) hotels.

The survey evidence, in particular, is drawn from a number of studies conducted at St Mary's Hospital, Paddington, since that part of London contains the largest concentration of B&B hotels used as temporary accommodation. The presence of large numbers of people in such hotels allowed epidemiological investigations with sufficient statistical power to identify significant differences between B&B dwellers and other population groups.

Though the people studied in London differ in some respects (for example in having a high proportion from ethnic minority groups) from other populations found in this accommodation type, in other more important respects (income, social class, household type, age) they resemble them. The findings from these studies are therefore likely to be applicable more widely and are useful pointers for designing local needs assessment work.

A different but more important problem is the lack of any systematic literature on the health effects of different types of temporary accommodation. This is particularly pertinent when assessing the likely influence of living for short periods of time in privately leased accommodation. At present there are only a few relevant studies but they indicate that health problems caused by housing conditions and housing status are not confined to those in B&B accommodation.

Families with children or pregnant women constituted 75% of the households accepted by local authorities as officially homeless in 1992.[1] There has been a massive increase in the number of officially accepted homeless households in recent years (Chapter 1). Many local authorities place most of these households in temporary accommodation because there is insufficient permanent housing available or, in some cases, in order to 'weed out' bogus applicants.[2]

Local authorities frequently use B&B hotels to provide short-term temporary accommodation for homeless families. In London as many as 60–70% of the placements are outside the accepting borough, resulting in isolation of families in unfamiliar neighbourhoods. The standard of accommodation in many of these hotels has been described by the Audit Commission as 'totally unsuited to family life'.[2] Recently, in London, more use has been made of privately leased and publicly owned accommodation on a temporary basis instead of B&B accommodation. Elsewhere the use of B&B appears to have levelled off.

There is little information on the characteristics of people who are accepted as homeless,[3] but a representative survey of homeless households placed in B&B hotels around Paddington[4] showed that:

• most adults were young, with 72% aged between 16 and 34 years, and only 2% over 65 years old;

• 79% had dependent children, and the majority had a single child of pre-school age;

• most people were from ethnic minority groups (35% were black, 30% were white from the UK; only 56% spoke English at home as their first language; some were political refugees);

• 72% had resided in the hotel for less than 6 months, but 5% had been there for more than 1 year;

• only 15% were in gainful employment; 54% were in receipt of income support; the main reasons for households becoming homeless were a breakdown of relationships, overcrowding and financial problems.

Two main aspects of the relationship between this type of homelessness and health have been studied — health status and health service utilisation.

HEALTH STATUS STUDIES

Housing conditions influence both physical and mental health and the assessment of this interrelationship is problematic.[5] The health of some people may be poor before they become homeless, especially political refugees and those recently arrived from abroad.

Most of the initial reports on the relatively poor health status of homeless households in B&B hotels were based on case reports by health visitors and other health professionals,[6–9] and by housing policy commentators.[10,11] They draw attention to the difficulty of trying to maintain good hygiene while living, washing, eating and sleeping in one overcrowded room. They report high levels of infections in the children, particularly gastroenteritis, skin disorders and chest infections, which may be related to overcrowding and poor hygiene. The children's diet was reported to be poor because of lack of money, poor knowledge about nutrition, and absent or inadequate kitchen facilities which force families to rely on food from cafes and take-aways. Normal child development is reported as impaired through lack of space for safe play and exploration. High rates of accidents to children are reported due to lack of space and hazards such as kettles at floor level.[12,13]

Social isolation, loneliness, boredom and loss of self-esteem contribute to the stress felt by the parents, and adversely affect their relationships with each other and their children.[11,14] Increased rates of behavioural problems in the children and delayed development are noted. Frequent changes of school not only disrupt a child's education but bring insecurity from repeated breaks in relation-ships and the need to adjust repeatedly to new and strange school environments. A report by HM Inspectorate of Schools on the edu-cation of children living in temporary accommodation drew atten-tion to the fact that some children have to join a waiting list before they can attend a local school, making future integration into new schools even more difficult.[15]

In addition to these reports by health professionals, a number of surveys have been carried out.[4,11,16]

Oxford survey

According to a survey of homeless families ($n = 47$) in Oxford,[16] many parents (46%) felt that their child's health had deteriorated since moving into B&B hotel accommodation (37% said it was the same, 7% better and 15% didn't know). Specific health problems were very poor sleeping (47%) and major eating problems (33%). For most families (80%) the bedroom was the only place for the child to play. Only 11% of the children aged under 5 years attended nursery or playgroup and 23% participated in a mother and toddler group. Parents reported that they felt tired most of the time (68%), were unhappy (60%), often could not sleep at night (58%), often lost their temper (65%) and were irritated by their child (55%). Their social isolation was demonstrated by the fact that 42% of those interviewed had spent eight or more waking hours in the bed-room during the previous day. Most families relied on cooking in their own bedroom (72%), often with nowhere suitable to prepare food. The health visitor who conducted the interviews felt that in only 2% of cases was the accommodation a safe and healthy

environment, while 85% were classified as very unsafe and unhealthy.

Parkside survey

More recently, a survey compared 319 homeless families with a
sample of local inner-city residents in Parkside District Health
Authority, London, and other residents of North West Thames
Region.[4] The regional health and lifestyle survey was administered
by trained interviewers. Of those who were homeless, 72% were
16–34 years old, compared with 31–33% of those permanently
resident.

Long-term physical illness. Almost half (46%) of the homeless people
reported that they had a long-term illness or disability lasting more
than a year. When the definition of chronic illness was confined to
problems that limit daily activity this was reduced to 34%. When
age-standardised against the North West Thames population
(standardised reference population = 100), it was found that these
problems were twice as common as in the housed population
(standardised limiting illness ratio = 205).

Acute illness. Homeless people reported higher rates of acute illness
in the previous 14 days than comparable age groups in the housed
population.

Mental health. Mental health status was measured with a 12-item
General Health Questionnaire. Significant mental morbidity was
shown in 45% of homeless people compared with 18–20% of local
or regional residents. The study did not try to identify major mental
disorder, although 4% of the B&B population as opposed to 1% of
the local residents were described as 'mentally ill'.

Adults living in temporary accommodation were found to present
more often with psychiatric problems to the local accident and
emergency department than local residents.[17] It is likely that most of
this mental morbidity is due to neurotic disorder. The high prevalence of mental morbidity amongst people in temporary accommodation may be related to uncertainty about the future, poor housing
conditions or overcrowding, as well as to predisposing factors such
as unemployment, social isolation, several dependent children or
recent adverse life events. The increased mental morbidity of
parents is likely to have an adverse effect on their children's
development.

Health behaviour. Smoking rates were significantly higher among homeless people than in the regional population (43% vs 21%), giving an age-standardised ratio of 156. Regular alcohol consumption was much lower amongst the homeless adults (45% vs 74%). Fewer homeless people participated in vigorous exercise; the age-standardised exercise ratio was 72. The diets of homeless people were much less likely than those of the regional comparison group to contain daily intakes of fresh fruit or vegetables (41% vs 57% and 44% vs 64% respectively).

Preventive health behaviour. Rates of cervical smear uptake were similar in the B&B homeless women and in the regional sample; 65% and 63% respectively of women aged 20–64 reported that they had had a cervical smear in the previous five years. Mothers' reports of completed courses of child immunisations amongst the B&B sample were fewer than in the regional comparison group: polio (85% homeless vs 87% region), diphtheria (74% vs 86%), tetanus (74% vs 84%), pertussis (74% vs 77%), measles (73% vs 82%).

St Mary's Hospital case-control study

In a separate investigation, designed as a prospective case-control study, conducted at St Mary's Hospital, London, acute medical admissions of children to the wards from B&B hotels during a 1-year period (*n* = 70) were compared with a control sample of admitted locally resident children.[18] A higher proportion of children from temporary accommodation had mild illnesses, though three of the B&B children died of overwhelming infections compared with none of the controls. A research health visitor interviewed each child's parents soon after discharge from hospital. Three times as many B&B mothers were depressed as those in permanent housing (24% vs 8%). The mothers had also experienced twice as many major life events in the previous year. The main complaints about the accommodation of the B&B mothers compared with the control mothers were:

- lack of space (70% vs 54%)
- nowhere safe for the children to play (68% vs 14%)
- isolation (58% vs 32%)
- noise (38% vs 30%)
- lack of privacy (32% vs 14%).

The health visitor assessed that only 2% of placements had

satisfactory play facilities, compared with 96% of locally resident children.

HEALTH SERVICE UTILISATION STUDIES

Victor and colleagues[17] reported significantly higher rates of hospital use among homeless people in B&B hotels in inner London. They estimated that the inpatient admission rate was 4.5 times greater than that for the resident population. For children, the hospital admission rate was more than twice that for the resident population. Overall, 9% of all acute, unplanned admissions at St Mary's Hospital, Paddington, were accounted for by people living in temporary B&B accommodation. The attendance rate at the paediatric emergency clinic in the hospital for children under 5 years of age was nearly twice that for local children. Homeless children were significantly more likely to attend with infectious diseases, and they had twice the accident rate for burns and scalds.[19]

The more recent survey conducted in Parkside DHA, London, showed a high rate of hospital and community health service utilisation (Table 3.1). Most (92%) families were registered with a general practitioner, but for a fifth of them the practice was over 8 km away. Special primary care services are provided for homeless families in the locality.

PREGNANCY

Patterson and Roderick studied outcome in homeless women (*n* = 185) attending St Mary's Hospital, London, in 1987–88.[20] Compared with local housed pregnant women there was a higher proportion of young women, women of high parity and those of Indo-Pakistani ethnicity (Table 3.2). Homeless women booked later and had had more previous obstetric problems than housed women. There were more preterm deliveries in the B&B women (11%) and the locally housed women (9%) than in the region as a whole (7%). When homeless women were matched for age, parity and ethnic origin with the local housed population, there was no difference in obstetric complications, intrapartum performance and perinatal outcome, though this may reflect the high levels of deprivation in the locally housed women and the high standard of obstetric care they received. Another study carried out in the east end of London found that 25% of babies born to mothers who had

TABLE 3.1   **Service utilisation (%) by homeless (B&B) people and housed comparison groups**

	Homeless		Parkside		NWTRHA	
	n	(%)	*n*	(%)	*n*	(%)
Consulted GP in previous 14 days	93	(29)	89	(16)	1568	(19)
Seen health visitor in previous 14 days	13	(4)	5	(1)	82	(1)
Visited casualty department in previous 14 days	42	(13)	17	(3)	2912	(5)
Visited outpatients in previous 3 months	38	(12)	66	(12)	1073	(13)
Hospital inpatient in previous 12 months (excluding obstetrics)	42	(13)	55	(10)	742	(9)
Visited NHS dentist in previous 14 days	19	(6)	44	(8)	577	(7)
n	*319*		*554*		*8251*	

Source: Victor CR. *A survey of the health status of the temporarily homeless population and residents of North West Thames Regional Health Authority.* Parkside Health Authority, 1992. (Ref 4)
Note: Parkside and NWTRHA data relate to all ages; the homeless sample data relate to a younger age group.

moved into B&B hotels in Hackney during pregnancy had birth-weights below 2,500g, compared with 10% amongst babies of local area resident mothers and about 7.2% in England.[9] This is disturbing, not only because of the relation of low birthweight to infant mortality but also, more speculatively, because of the relationship of growth retardation to the child's cardiovascular risk in adult life.[21]

TABLE 3.2   **Demographic characteristics of homeless and housed pregnant women**

	No. (%) of homeless women (n = 185)	No. (%) of housed women (n = 2123)
Ethnic group:[a]		
African	16 (9)	125 (6)
White	64 (35)	1196 (56)
Indo-Pakistani	74 (40)	194 (9)
West Indian	14 (8)	266 (13)
Other	17 (9)	342 (16)
Parity:[b]		
0	54 (29)	1036 (49)
1–3	86 (46)	992 (47)
≥4	45 (24)	95 (4)
Maternal age at delivery:[c]		
<20	24 (13)	103 (5)
20–24	52 (28)	493 (23)
25–29	37 (20)	657 (31)
30–34	47 (25)	523 (25)
≥35	25 (14)	347 (16)

[a]$\chi^2 = 164.9$, df 4, p < 0.001.
[b]$\chi^2 = 110.9$, df 2, p < 0.001.
[c]$\chi^2 = 29.8$, df 4, p < 0.001.
Source: Table I: Patterson CM, Roderick PJ. *BMJ* 1990; **301**: 263–6. (Ref 20)

RECOMMENDATION 4

Health commissioning authorities should assess the health and health care needs of members of homeless households and should commission services to meet these needs.

RECOMMENDATION 5

Health Authorities and Family Health Service Authorities should ensure that members of homeless households placed in temporary accommodation have access to full registration with a local general practitioner.

References to Chapter 3 appear on page 128.

4 The health of single homeless people

SUMMARY

- Although there are methodological problems with most of the studies of the health of single homeless people, the accumulated results present a clear picture of their health status.

- Single homeless people experience higher levels of mortality and morbidity than housed people.

- The results of studies in the UK, Sweden and the USA are largely consistent with each other.

- Excess mortality is due mainly to deaths from violence, suicide, accidents, alcohol-related diseases and respiratory disorders.

- Single homeless people experience higher levels of physical illness across a broad range of conditions. Excess rates of respiratory, gastrointestinal, musculoskeletal, dermatological and neurological disorders are recorded. Specific conditions that are over-represented include tuberculosis, chronic obstructive airways disease, trauma, foot problems, infestations and epilepsy.

- Tuberculosis represents a special problem because of difficulties with treatment compliance, which can result in the emergence of drug-resistant strains of *Mycobacterium tuberculosis* which may spread into the general population and so constitute a threat to public health.

- Single homeless people have high rates of alcohol and drug misuse.

- There are high levels of mental disorder among single homeless people (see Chapter 5).

- The high levels of illness among single homeless people can be explained by:

  - poor health causing homelessness (see Chapter 2)
  - poor health produced by homelessness
  - poor health prolonged or exacerbated by homelessness.

'When I moved into _____ and I was getting regular dinners, and do you know I was six months ill through all this. It hurts because your system can't cope with it. You're having proper hot dinners.'

'I'm starting Youth Training, and I'm positive I'm gonna get myself sorted out.'

'I will probably die somewhere in a shop doorway.'[65]

INTRODUCTION

The subject of this chapter is the health of single homeless people (Group II) who are not included among the 'official' homeless. We first consider methodological problems and then present two sections relating to physical disease and disability, and substance abuse disorders. An attempt is made to answer two questions:

- What is the evidence that the health of the single homeless population is *worse* than that of comparable housed populations?
- Why are certain disorders *over-represented* amongst single homeless people?

METHODOLOGICAL PROBLEMS

It is not easy to assess the evidence for an *excessive* level of particular diseases or disabilities among single homeless people, compared with a housed population of similar age and gender. Most of the United Kingdom studies are on a small scale and they vary in sampling, data-gathering procedures, item validation, diagnostic classifications, analyses and presentation of results. Moreover, the available studies span nearly three decades, during which time the causes of homelessness and consequently the socio-demographic characteristics of those becoming homeless have changed significantly. It is also difficult to define an appropriate population group to compare with Group II homeless people.

The shortcomings of the available UK data mean that on occasions it has been necessary to refer to studies from abroad, particularly from the USA. Such studies must, however, be interpreted with caution.

Table 4.1 summarises studies of the health of single homeless people (Group II). These studies may be classified according to four characteristics: (i) sample selection; (ii) data collection techniques; (iii) use of comparison groups; (iv) whether the study deals with mortality or morbidity.

(i) Sample selection

A study of single homeless people that sought to estimate the prevalence of specific diseases would ideally be based on a suitable large sample that was representative of the whole group. Unfortunately it is difficult and costly to obtain such *representative* samples. Most UK studies are based on samples of homeless people in particular settings. Some studies have described patients presenting for treatment to special GP clinics in hostels or other temporary accommodation. Others have surveyed people living in a particular hostel. Such samples, whilst convenient for research purposes, may result in findings that are prone to selection bias. For example, if the sample is based on consultations there may be a bias towards finding high rates of morbidity because those who consult are usually in poorer health than those who do not.

(ii) Data collection techniques

An ideal study of the health of homeless people would include standardised examinations and suitable physical investigations. Unfortunately there are few studies that approach this ideal. Most UK studies rely on data collected retrospectively from the case notes of GPs and other primary health care workers, and hence they require cautious interpretation. Another important problem is the underdetection of disorders amongst homeless people seen only once by a doctor.[1] This potential bias would tend to reduce reported differences between Group II homeless people and housed consulter populations, because the latter are likely to be better known to their doctors and so more likely to have their diseases diagnosed.

(iii) Use of comparison groups

An ideal study of the health of homeless people would make use of a suitable comparison group. Many authors of studies on homeless people believe that their results 'speak for themselves'. They

TABLE 4.1 **Studies of the pattern of disease amongst Group II homeless people**

Study setting	GP clinic attenders	Population sample (self-report)	Population sample (with examination)	Mortality study
(a) UK studies				
Used comparison group	Shanks 1988[1]; Balazs 1992[3]	George 1991[5] Whynes 1992[4] Bines 1994[2]	Lodge-Patch 1971[6] Featherstone 1988[7]	Shanks 1984 Keyes 1992
No comparison group	Morrell 1966; Scott 1966; Gaskell 1969; Shanks 1983; Powell 1987; Toon 1987; Braddick 1989; Ramsden 1989			
(b) Selected studies from abroad				
Used comparison group	HCH 1987		Breakey 1989[8]	Alstrom 1975
No comparison group				—

[1]Compared observed number of consultations for each diagnosis with expected levels in the general population with adjustment for social class.

[2]Compared frequency of self-reported symptoms with data from the British Household Panel Survey; sample is probably representative of the Group II homeless population.

[3]Compared proportion of consultations for each diagnosis with expected proportion for the general population: sample is probably not representative of the Group II homeless population.

[4]Compared frequency of self-reported health problems to data from the General Household Survey; sample is probably representative of the Group II homeless population.

[5]Compared responses on the Nottingham Health Profile to normative data from housed population.

[6]Sample restricted to hostel dwellers.

[7]Sample restricted to hostel dwellers.

[8]Based on representative sample of Group II homeless.

consider that the prevalences of diseases observed are obviously larger than would be expected in the general (housed) population. Although this assumption is justified for some disorders, for others the influence of age, sex and social class is important and it is crucial to compare reported prevalence rates with the appropriate comparison group. Moreover, to *quantify* any reported excess (or deficit) of a disorder, a comparison group must be used.

(iv)   Whether the study deals with mortality or morbidity

An ideal study of the health of homeless people would take account of both mortality and morbidity. Studies of mortality amongst homeless people are valuable pointers to the general health of the homeless population. However, such studies tend to be influenced by the administrative rules and procedures used in categorising cause of death. For example, deaths due to alcohol-related diseases such as cirrhosis of the liver and pancreatitis tend to be under-reported in known alcoholics. Suicide is also under-reported because in most countries, including the UK, this is a medico-legal classification which may be made only if certain evidence is available. Moreover, studies of mortality alone tell us nothing of the disability and suffering caused by disorders not directly linked to the cause of death.

In summary, an ideal study of the health of homeless people would: (i) be based on a representative sample; (ii) include a clinical examination; (iii) make use of a suitable comparison group; and (iv) consider both mortality and morbidity. From Table 4.1 it can be seen that there have been no ideal studies of the health of homeless people in the UK. Out of the seven studies that used comparison groups, three are based on self-report only, whilst two deal exclusively with mortality. The remaining two studies are based on an unrepresentative sample (GP clinic attenders) and take into account only presenting diagnosis. In the light of these methodological limitations, the interpretation of results from any individual study must be treated cautiously.

PHYSICAL DISORDERS

Studies of mortality amongst homeless people will be discussed first, followed by morbidity studies. In each case UK studies will be discussed first, and will then be supplemented by further data from selected studies from outside the UK.

Studies of mortality

Studies from the United Kingdom

An early UK study showed that the proportion of deaths from cancer and respiratory diseases (including tuberculosis) amongst residents of a common lodging house was higher than that in the general population, but the proportion of deaths from heart disease and stroke was lower.[2] However, since that study looked at proportional mortality rates in the two groups, rather than comparing absolute rates, it was inevitable that if some rates were higher others would be compensatingly lower.

More recently, Keyes and colleagues carried out a study of inner London coroner's court records for the period from September 1991 to August 1992.[3] Decedents who were homeless and conformed to the definition of Group II (Chapter 1) were identified, and death rates were compared with those expected in an age-matched general population. Group II homeless people accounted

TABLE 4.2   **Deaths and excess mortality amongst Group II homeless people 1991–92, by cause of death**

Cause	Average age (years)	Observed	O/E[a]
Accidents	51	16	7.7
Assault/murder	38	6	156.3
Pneumonia or hypothermia	54	11	2.9
Other natural causes	66	15	NA
Not known	43	3	NA
Drug overdose	34	11	30.2
Alcohol poisoning	45	4	16.9
Suicide	37	20	33.6
Total	*47*	*86*	*2.8*

Source: Keyes S, Kennedy M. *Sick to death of homelessness.* London: Crisis, December 1992. (Ref 3)
NA = Not available
[a]Calculated by grossing up observed deaths to obtain a national death rate amongst the single homeless, assuming London comprises 38% of English total, and dividing this rate by the rate amongst the general population.

for 86 deaths (82% male, average age 47). The total mortality was 2.8 times that expected; cause-specific mortality is shown in Table 4.2. The authors of this study argue that their method of ascertaining deaths is likely to have biased their results so that, overall, there would be an underestimate of 'natural' deaths amongst Group II homeless people (due, for example, to missing deaths occurring in hospital), while deaths due to 'unnatural' causes would be less liable to this bias. The findings of this study are largely in agreement with those of overseas studies.

Studies from the United States

Three US studies describe the age, gender and ethnicity of decedents, and allow the calculation of crude all-cause mortality rates and proportional mortality ratios for particular disorders.[1,4,5] In Atlanta, Georgia, from July 1985 to June 1986, 40 deaths occurred among homeless people. The median age at death was 43 for black men (48% of deaths) and 53 for white men (45%). Deaths were classified as natural (the consequence of a disease or of the ageing process) (40%), accidental (unintentional) (48%), homicide (10%) and suicide (2%); 70% of all deaths were alcohol-related.[4]

In a larger study in San Francisco, California, in 1985–90, 644 deaths were identified; 88% were men (68% white, 24% black, 4% Hispanic, 2% American Indian/Alaskan). The average age at death was 41 years (standard deviation ±12 years). Using the same broad classification scheme as in the Atlanta study, 39% of deaths were natural, 34% were due to unintentional (accidental) injuries, 13% resulted from homicide, 6% from suicide and 9% from undetermined cause. Alcohol was present in the blood of 47% of decedents, and 34% had levels above 100 mg/dl. Morphine (the breakdown product of heroin) was detected in 21%, and there was evidence that illicit drug use amongst decedents increased from 27% in 1985 to 46% in 1990.[5]

The third US study has been reported by Wright and Weber who also give seven illustrative case histories of the circumstances leading up to death.[1] The methods used in this study did not allow reliable estimates of crude death rates. However, a calculation for a selected sub-population (those who had three or more consultations during a year and were still in contact with the program at the time of death) gave a rate amongst the homeless people (737 per 100,000) that was 3.1 times the prevailing general US death rate. The median age at death was 51 years.

A recent study from Philadelphia confirms these findings and reports a death rate among homeless people 3.5 times that of the general population.[6]

A study from Sweden

In a study from Sweden a more sophisticated approach was used.[7] Alstrom *et al* used systematically collected records of 6,032 men registered in Stockholm at the bureau for homeless men from 1969 to 1971 and matched them to death certificates from the Swedish central bureau of statistics. The results showed that there was significant excess mortality for all age groups. This was especially striking among those aged under 40 and was observed in all diagnostic categories: accidents, poisonings and violence (12 times expected rates); suicide (×4); cirrhosis of the liver (×6); diseases of the digestive system (×7); diseases of the respiratory system (×7); pulmonary tuberculosis (×6); diseases of the circulatory system (×3); diseases of the nervous system and sense organs (×4); neoplasm (×2).

Studies of morbidity

Studies from the United Kingdom

The characteristics of the UK studies are summarised in Table 4.1. These studies are useful if taken together, but each falls short of the ideal in design and analysis. The results must therefore be treated with caution, and further analysis and interpretation will necessitate the inclusion of studies from the United States.

Of the five studies that used comparison groups, that by George *et al*, being a census of 340 single homeless people from sites in Sheffield identified as places of residence of homeless people, is likely to be fairly representative for the Group II homeless population.[8] Although the data were largely based on self-reports and so are of limited value in estimating the prevalence of specific disorders, the study showed that homeless people perceived their health as significantly worse than that of a comparable housed population on all dimensions of the Nottingham Health Profile.

The larger national survey by Bines was also based on self-reports of symptoms.[9] A representative sample of 1,346 homeless people interviewed across the UK was divided into three groups: subjects living in hostels or B&B (*n* = 1,280), those using day centres (*n* = 351) and those using soup runs (*n* = 156). The second and third groups consisted of rough sleepers. The responses of the subjects, for specific categories of symptoms, were compared with data from the British Household Panel Survey, carried out during the same year. Although the data from this study cannot be used to calculate the prevalence of specific disorders, they nevertheless indicate that a representative sample of homeless people report certain symptoms more commonly than a representative sample of the housed population.

The study by Whynes and Giggs was also based on self-report data.[10] The survey was of approximately 2,000 subjects applying for accommodation to statutory and voluntary agencies in Nottingham. Subjects were asked whether they had any health problems and the numbers reporting problems were then compared with findings from the General Household Survey in Nottingham. Unusually, the homeless people had significantly fewer mental and physical problems than the housed population, but this finding is probably due to two problems in analysis: the two groups were not matched by age (the homeless group was much younger than the housed group), and a large proportion of the homeless people were in either Group I or Group III, so it is not possible to establish how far the findings can be applied to people in Group II.

The remaining studies that used a comparison group are those by Shanks[11] and by Balazs.[12] Both studies compared the consultation rates of homeless patients with those of a general population sample matched for social class. Shanks found that overall consultation rates were not higher among homeless people, though he observed high rates for psychiatric and dermatological conditions and low rates for cardiovascular and musculoskeletal conditions. It is difficult to assess total morbidity from this study because only the presenting diagnosis was recorded, so there is no information about coexisting health problems. Moreover, consultation rates alone are only an indirect indicator of health and are subject to many influences other than acute levels of morbidity.

In the more recent study by Balazs[12] of 2,200 consultations with GPs working with the HHELP team in east London, consultation rates were compared with expected rates for housed patients of similar socio-economic status, derived from the morbidity statistics for general practice. This study, which had similar methodological limitations to that of Shanks, found that homeless people had significantly more consultations for cardiovascular, dermatological and musculoskeletal problems than the housed group.

All the remaining UK studies are based on samples unlikely to be representative of the Group II population. They involved selected samples either of attenders at special clinics for homeless people[13-19] or of those living in hostels for homeless people.[20-22] It is important to emphasise that these studies show only how often particular groups of disorders present to doctors who work in special clinics. They are not population based studies and cannot demonstrate differences in morbidity between housed and homeless people. The only exception is where disorders known to be rare in the general population are reported frequently in the special GP clinics.

Table 4.3 summarises the findings of these studies and shows that respiratory, musculoskeletal and dermatological disorders are common amongst clinic attenders. As these disorders are also common in ordinary GP clinics, we cannot simply assume that they are *excessively* prevalent amongst the homeless population. However, the very high frequency of tuberculosis (mean 9.6% of attenders) implies that it is more common amongst homeless people.

Non-UK studies

The existing UK studies may be interpreted in the light of studies from other countries on the extent and level of morbidity among single homeless people. Reliable estimates of excess prevalence of specific disorders are not available from UK studies and therefore we have used studies from other developed industrialised countries to indicate:

• the likely level of excess morbidity among the UK homeless population compared with the housed population;

• the disorders that are more likely to be over-represented amongst the UK homeless population.

US studies

Two American studies are considered to be particularly useful. In a study in Baltimore that used a large representative sample, with standardised examinations, but had no comparison group, 528 homeless people were randomly selected from a baseline survey of the missions, shelters and jails.[23] Half were randomly allocated to receive standardised physical and psychiatric examinations and 195 subjects were assessed. Clinical examinations were accompanied by an electrocardiogram, a chest X-ray, haematology screening tests, liver function tests, urinalysis, screening for gonorrhoea, tuberculin skin test, and stool examination for intestinal parasites. Health problems were recorded if they were considered by the examining physician to be worthy of the attention of a primary care provider. The findings show high levels of dermatological, dental, cardiovascular and respiratory problems.

A number of lessons about the UK population can be drawn from the Baltimore study:

  i the health of unselected samples of homeless people may be as bad or even worse than that of homeless people seen in GP clinics;

TABLE 4.3   **Studies of physical disorder amongst single homeless people, showing percentage with specific disorders**

Disorder	Gaskell	Shanks	Powell	Ramsden[a]	Toon	Scott[b]	Braddick	Lodge-Patch	Balazs	Bines c	Bines d	Bines e
Respiratory	16.50	13.70	22.40	27.40	17	17.50	10	9	17.4	18	24	28
Musculoskeletal	22.70	10.50	3.60	30.82	16	8.40	NR	5	9.1	12	27	30
Dermatological	7.60	6.10	9.30	22.60	28	NR	24	1	21.8	10	16	20
Gastrointestinal	7.00	7.30	11.80	8.90	11	NR	6	NR	9.9	8	13	13
Cardiovascular	6.30	3.80	8.10	4.79	NR	4.80	NR	5	4.2	5	6	5
Neurological and epilepsy	4.60	NR	4.30	6.85	4	7.20	NR	11	4.3	16	18	20
Carcinoma	2.90	0.70	2.50	NR	NR	4.40	NR	NR	NR	NR	NR	NR
Orodental	NR	NR	NR	NR	2	NR	NR	NR	NR	NR	NR	NR
Genitourinary	NR	NR	NR	1.37	NR	NR	NR	NR	NR	5	6	6
Tubercular	NR	NR	NR	3.40	15	11.90	NR	8	NR	NR	NR	NR

NR = not reported.
[a]Mobile GP clinic.
[b]Based on sample at common lodging house.
[c]Hostel and B&B survey.
[d]Day Centre survey.
[e]Soup-run survey.

ii the UK homeless population are also likely to have multiple disorders;

iii the rates of dermatological, respiratory and musculoskeletal disorders reported in UK studies may reflect a high and *excessive* frequency of these disorders in the homeless population as a whole, rather than be due to sampling bias.

The Health Care of the Homeless (HCH) program brought together data from 19 primary health care programs for homeless people in 19 American cities.[1] Data on the health of 23,745 homeless adults have been reported. This study is not based on a representative sample of homeless people, data are not based on standardised examinations, and most of the data on disease prevalence refer to patients who attended a clinic on more than one occasion. The study may therefore overestimate the prevalence of physical disorders.

Despite these limitations, the HCH data are of considerable value in assessing the UK studies because they provide an estimate of the extent to which particular disorders may be over-represented. Table 4.4 lists the disorders that the HCH study found to be most over-represented amongst homeless people. These include: infestations (49 times more common than in housed populations); dental problems (×31); peripheral vascular disease (×14.5); sexually transmitted diseases (STD) (×8); tuberculosis (×5); minor respiratory tract infections (×5); neurological disorders (×6); liver disease (×4.3); gastrointestinal disorders (×2.5); haematological disorders (×2.4); genitourinary disorders common to both men and women (×2.3); genitourinary disorders of women (×2.2); syphilis (×2). It is not possible to calculate the relative occurrence of trauma, although analyses of individual types of trauma suggest that it is also over-represented.

Comparison of US studies and European studies*

The US studies are compared with European studies in Table 4.4. A disorder is considered to be over-represented among homeless people in the UK studies if any of the following conditions are fulfilled:

i the authors comment that a particular disorder appears to be over-represented in its sample;

---

*The studies from the US are here considered together with the study by Alstrom.

ii there is a reported prevalence of more than 2% for a disorder known to be rare in the housed population (<0.5%
prevalence);

iii the study has found the disorder to be a cause of death amongst
homeless people more frequently than would be expected in the
housed population;

iv the disorder is reported to be significantly more common among
homeless people than among a comparable group of housed
patients.

Agreement between the US and European studies is assessed as:

good — more than four European studies concordant with
US findings

fair — three or four European studies concordant with US
findings

poor — less than three European studies concordant with
US findings.

According to these criteria, there is good or fair agreement between
US and UK studies that the following general categories of disorder
are over-represented: respiratory (7 studies); dermatological (5
studies); musculoskeletal (3 studies); gastrointestinal (4 studies);
neurological (3 studies). Within these broad categories there is
good agreement that tuberculosis (10 studies), trauma (7 studies)
and epilepsy (6 studies) are over-represented, and fair agreement
that chronic bronchitis (3 studies), foot problems (3 studies) and
infestations (4 studies) are over-represented.

There is disagreement between US and UK studies on the following points. First, three UK studies assert that neoplasms are over-
represented, but this is not supported by the US data. Second, UK
studies do not agree that orodental, genitourinary, haematological,
cardiovascular and liver disorders, arthritis and pneumonia are
over-represented. It seems likely from the recent work of Featherstone *et al*[22] and Balazs[12] that orodental disorders are probably
under-reported in the UK literature because GPs do not routinely
check dental hygiene. Similarly, it is possible that genitourinary disorders are under-reported.

There are insufficient data from the US studies to compare the
prevalence of HIV infection in the US homeless population with
that in the housed population. However, US studies restricted to
estimating the prevalence of HIV amongst homeless people suggest
that it is common. No information is available on the prevalence of
HIV in the UK homeless population.

TABLE 4.4   **Agreement between European and selected American studies**

	US studies		European studies					
			Mortality studies (odds)					
Disorder	HCH (odds)	Breakey[a] (%)	Keyes (1992)	Alstrom (1975)	Shanks (1984)	Scott (1966)	Morrell (1967)	Gaskell (1969)
RESPIRATORY								
▶ Overall	×3.9	40		×7	×3.4	yes	yes	
Pneumonia	—	—	×2.9					
Minor	×5	—						
▶ Tuberculosis	×5	—		×6		yes	yes	
▶ COAD[c]	—	—				yes	yes	
MUSCULO-SKELETAL								
▶ Overall	—	38						
▶ Trauma	×2.9	—	×7.7	×12	×1.3	yes	yes	
▶ Feet	—	—						
Arthritis	×1.1	26						
DERMATOLOGICAL								
▶ Overall	×3.1	58						
▶ Infestations	×49	—						
GASTRO-INTESTINAL								
▶ Overall	×2.5	—		×7				
Liver	×4.3	—		×6				
CARDIOVASCULAR								
Overall	×1.1	52.5		×3				
NEUROLOGICAL[d]								
▶ Overall	×6.2	33		×4				
▶ Epilepsy	—	—				yes	yes	yes
NEOPLASTIC								
Overall	—	—		×2	yes	yes		
ORODENTAL								
Overall	×31	68						
GENITO-URINARY								
Overall	×2.3	—						
STD[e]	×8	8						
Gynae	—	64						
HAEMATOLOGICAL								
Overall	×2.4	—						
Anaemia	—	18.3						

▶ Indicates good or fair agreement between US and UK studies (see text for a full explanation).
[a]Data was reported separately for males and females, for maximum comparability with other studies. Data for males is reported here, except for gynaecological problems, overall genito-urinary and STD. Anaemia was more common in homeless women (34.7%), but otherwise there were no striking gender differences in the study.

European studies

Morbidity studies

Lodge-Patch (1971)	Shanks (1983)	Powell (1987)	Toon (1987)	Shanks (1988)	Feather-stone (1988)	Braddick (1989)	Ramsden (1989)	George (1991)	Balazs (1992)	Bines (1994)	N[b]
		yes					yes			yes	7
									yes		2
											0
yes	yes	yes	yes				yes	yes			9
					yes						3
							yes		yes	yes	3
			yes		yes						7
			yes		yes				yes		3
							yes				1
	yes			yes	yes				yes	yes	5
			yes			yes	yes		yes		4
		yes	yes							yes	4
											1
									yes		2
			yes							yes	3
yes		yes			yes						6
											3
					yes				yes		2
			yes								1
											0
											0
			yes								1
											0

[b] Number of UK/European studies in agreement. [c] COAD = chronic obstructive airways disease.
[d] Including head injuries. [e] STD = sexually transmitted disease.

REASONS FOR INCREASED LEVELS OF DISEASE AMONG HOMELESS PEOPLE

The preceding section has shown that certain disorders are more commonly found among homeless than among housed people. The reasons for the high prevalence of physical disorders among homeless people may be summarised as follows:

1. Physical disorders are associated with becoming homeless

Pre-existing physical disorders may impair a person's ability to earn money and hence to find and keep accommodation, and so can lead to homelessness. In the absence of effective social policies, disabling physical disorders would be likely to be over-represented among homeless people. A general argument for the link between health and homelessness is discussed in detail in Chapter 2.

2. Physical disorders are produced by homelessness

Once homeless, an individual is at risk of developing new physical disorders as a result of the lack of adequate shelter, privacy, sanitation, security and an inadequate diet. Lack of shelter results in exposure to inclement weather and increases the risk of accidents. Lack of privacy increases exposure to infectious diseases in large communal dwellings. Lack of sanitation leads to disorders associated with poor personal hygiene. Lack of security increases the chance of violent attack and rape. Lack of an adequate diet results in malnutrition and reduced immunity to disease.[24,25]

3. Physical disorders are maintained and exacerbated by homelessness

Pre-existing disorders and new disorders may be maintained or exacerbated by homelessness. The factors set out in the preceding paragraph which lead to disease are compounded by poor access to medical care (see Chapter 6) and difficulties in complying with treatment which may be due to inebriation, adverse environments, frequent change of 'address', and difficulties in obtaining and keeping appointments.

4. Physical disorder may be caused or exacerbated by behaviour associated with homelessness

Many homeless people behave in ways that tend to cause or exacerbate physical disorder. Underlying these behaviours, it may be argued, is a basic lack of concern for their long-term health prospects. This attitude, if present, is perhaps not surprising amongst people whose poor quality of life is often mitigated by health-damaging behaviour. A quotation from a homeless youth interviewed during an American study of HIV infection sums up this attitude: 'Why should I care about dying ten years from now, when I don't know where I will sleep and how I'll get food tomorrow?'[26]

There are three behaviours commonly associated with homelessness that are likely to affect health adversely: alcohol abuse, drug abuse and prostitution.

Alcohol abuse. The HCH study[1] showed that alcohol abuse appeared to have an adverse effect on health, over and above that attributable to homelessness. Chronic liver disease was 4.3 times more common among alcohol abusers than among other homeless people. Nutritional disorders, trauma, serious skin disorders and serious respiratory infections were substantially more common among the alcohol abusers, as were all chronic disorders except diabetes.

Substance abuse. Substance (drug) abusers were also in poorer health than homeless people who did not abuse drugs. HIV infection was 4.5 times more common amongst homeless drug abusers, and neurological dis-orders, anaemia, eye diseases, cardiac disease, chronic obstructive lung disease, sexually transmitted diseases, and other infectious disorders were significantly more common in homeless people who abused drugs.[1] It seems reasonable to assume that these findings also apply to UK homeless populations.

Prostitution. Little is known about the extent of prostitution in the UK homeless populations, although it is occasionally alluded to in the literature.[27] It is likely to be an option for survival on the streets, especially among young people.[28] The health-damaging consequences of prostitution include increased prevalence of HIV infection amongst young male prostitutes, reported in American surveys,[26] as well as other sexually transmitted diseases. Prostitutes are also at increased risk of violent assault.

SPECIFIC MEDICAL DISORDERS ASSOCIATED WITH HOMELESSNESS

This section will consider why particular disorders are over-represented amongst homeless people and will deal with those disorders for which there is good or fair agreement between US and UK studies (see Table 4.4).

Respiratory disorders

It is likely that many of the 'respiratory infections' reported in studies of homeless people refer to mild upper respiratory tract infections. However, pneumonia and/or pleurisy was diagnosed by Stephens *et al*[29] in about 3% of consultations with homeless people; this is three times the occurrence rate in the housed population. Pneumonia was diagnosed in 8% of homeless youths attending a medical clinic in the US.[26]

Homeless people seem to be at particular risk of pneumococcal pneumonia, as indicated by two recent reports of outbreaks of this disorder: during 1988–9 in Paris[30] and in Boston.[31] Both reports noted that epidemics of pneumococcal pneumonia, rare in the general population since the arrival of antibiotics, now tend to occur amongst residents of shelters for homeless people. Of the homeless people affected in the French outbreak, 60% developed bacteraemia compared with 25% in the general population, and the prognosis of homeless people appeared to be worse.

The high incidence of respiratory disorders amongst homeless people may be because many are heavy smokers. Studies from the US have shown that 73% of homeless people smoke, compared with 40% of poor housed people attending the same clinic.[32] Up to 93% of the homeless people in Oxford were smokers,[33] while the HHELP team in east London reported that 85% of their male patients and 73% of their female patients were smokers.[12] In the Baltimore study, all the homeless people who participated in medical examinations were heavy smokers, with 40% smoking more than 40 cigarettes per day.[23]

Tuberculosis

Tuberculosis has again become a clinical and public health problem, after a long period of declining incidence in developed countries.[34] There is now good evidence that the incidence of tuberculosis is increasing in the US;[35] for example, the number of reported cases of tuberculosis increased by 20% during 1985–90,[36] and 1990 saw the largest annual increase since 1953.[37] In Europe, tuberculosis is on the increase in Austria, Denmark, Ireland, Netherlands, Norway, Italy and Switzerland.[38] Compared to the US, the UK situation is less clear,[39] but recent figures show that since

1987 the raw number of cases in England and Wales has steadily increased; for example, notifications increased by 5% in 1992, and for the first four months of 1993 they showed a 7% increase on the equivalent period in 1992.[40,41]

Some commentators have attributed the rising incidence of tuberculosis in part to the rising numbers of homeless people.[42,43] This section will consider the relationship between homelessness and tuberculosis in terms of (i) the reasons why tuberculosis has tended to persist amongst homeless people, (ii) whether tuberculosis is now increasing amongst homeless people, and (iii) how far tuberculosis amongst homeless people is now posing a threat to the health of the general population.

(i) The persistence of tuberculosis amongst homeless people

The incidence of tuberculosis amongst homeless people never fell to the levels found in the general population in the latter part of this century.[34] Throughout the 1980s the disorder remained a significant cause of mortality and morbidity for homeless people. Thus in Manchester, during 1977–81, tuberculosis was the cause of 25% of all deaths due to respiratory diseases amongst homeless people,[2] whilst studies of attenders at clinics for homeless people in London reported a 15% lifetime prevalence of pulmonary tuberculosis, and a 0.82% incidence of active tuberculosis compared with 0.027% among the general housed population.[13,44]

The persistence of tuberculosis can be explained by four factors. First, homeless people are more likely to catch tuberculosis or to experience reactivation of old lesions owing to their generally poor state of health and nutrition.[45] Second, many homeless people spend time in overcrowded and poorly ventilated hostels where communal living conditions are ideal for the transmission of tuberculosis.[46] Third, a proportion of homeless people who contract tuberculosis do not comply with treatment and may move from hostel to hostel spreading the disorder. The reasons for this lack of compliance are not clear; in some cases it may be due to the patient's unsettled lifestyle.[47] Thus, homeless people are particularly likely to have difficulties complying with the necessary long-term multiple drug regime.[48,49] In other cases mental disorder or substance abuse has been implicated;[50] for example a study in east London showed a strong association between alcoholism and tuberculosis, in that 42% of patients admitted to a tuberculosis ward were dependent on alcohol, of whom 80% were homeless.[51]

Finally, the level of medical care available to most homeless people makes early detection and successful treatment of tuberculosis less likely. Even where care is good there are often delays in diagnosis and treatment. Capewell *et al*[52] highlighted the difficulties in diagnosis and management of tuberculosis, which are compounded where organisms are drug-resistant or where other infections such as *Pneumocystis carinii* are present.

(ii) Is tuberculosis increasing amongst homeless people?

Recently it has become clear that tuberculosis (including drug-resistant forms) is increasing amongst homeless people in certain parts of the US.[53] It is generally believed that a key factor has been the spread of HIV in this population.[53] For example, 18% of a group of homeless men requesting HIV testing in New York were found to have active tuberculosis.[54] Infection with HIV facilitates the spread of tuberculosis because immunocompromised people are more likely than other homeless people to become infected or to experience reactivation of old foci.

As yet there is no evidence that tuberculosis is on the increase amongst the homeless population in the UK,[34] but this may be because relevant data are not available. Levels of HIV infection amongst the homeless population in the UK are not known.

(iii) How far does tuberculosis amongst homeless people pose a threat to the health of the general population?

Rising levels of tuberculosis amongst homeless people in the US have been associated with rising levels in the general population. The question arises therefore as to whether rising levels in the homeless population may be responsible for rising levels in the general population. Although this question is difficult to answer for certain, it appears that tuberculosis amongst single homeless people poses two threats to public health. The disease tends to spread from homeless people to other groups within the general (housed) population and drug-resistant strains of tuberculosis tend to develop amongst homeless people.

Spread of tuberculosis from homeless people to other groups   A key factor in the resurgence of tuberculosis in the US has been the spread of HIV infection, which reduces immunity to *Mycobacterium tuberculosis*. In the UK at present only 5% of people with HIV are found to be suffering from tuberculosis, a level much lower than in comparable populations in the US.[55] This difference is said to reflect the small overlap between the population with HIV and those at risk of mycobacterial infection.[56] However, within the growing population of homeless people in the UK, there are increasing opportunities for overlap between those at risk of HIV infection (for example, intravenous drug users or workers in the sex industry) and those at risk of tuberculosis. Moreover, this overlap is likely to occur under conditions ideal for the transmission of tuberculosis — overcrowded and poorly ventilated hostels. Once tuberculosis becomes established amongst those at risk of HIV in the UK, further transmission to acquaintances, partners and children occurs, as described in reports from the US.[39]

Recently the application of new molecular biological techniques to epidemiology has demonstrated how marginalised groups, such as drug users and homeless people, are vulnerable to each other's infections, and how these infections may then be passed on to the general population.[53] A recent study of outbreaks of tuberculosis in Berne, using DNA 'fingerprinting' techniques, described the spread of a strain of tuberculosis amongst members of the local 'drug scene' and users of local hostels for the homeless.[43] The strain then spread to a waitress and owner of a local restaurant patronised by drug users. The origin of the outbreak was traced to a homeless alcoholic, first diagnosed in 1987, who complied poorly with anti-tuberculous treatment and who for some years had mixed freely with the community from which most of the 1991–2 cases came. The outbreak accounted for 13% of tuberculosis cases notified in the canton. The study concluded that: (i) active transmission of *M. tuberculosis* is now taking place in Europe in the same social milieu as in the US; (ii) there is a definite 'spillover' into the general population; and (iii) the dimensions of the problem are hard to assess because of the complex pattern of transmission. The authors called for 'concerted action at national and European levels' to control the spread of tuberculosis, and redefinition of 'high-risk groups', and the instituting of targeted treatment programs. This contrasts with recent proposals for the cessation of BCG vaccination programs for teenagers,[57] and with the reported closure of tuberculosis prevention programs by NHS Trusts.[58]

Development of multiple drug-resistant strains of tuberculosis amongst homeless people   Tuberculosis infections in homeless people are often drug-resistant.[47] For example, 50 out of 87 individuals suffering from isoniazid-resistant tuberculosis in Glasgow over the years 1981–8 were homeless.[48]

Drug resistance in tuberculosis is either primary or secondary; both types occur in homeless people. Primary resistance occurs when a person is infected with mycobacteria that have already acquired drug resistance. Secondary resistance occurs when previously non-resistant mycobacteria acquire resistance during treatment. This may be because the medication in inadequate or because the patient is failing to take the medication in the recommended way.[59]

The main reason for the high levels of drug-resistant tuberculosis amongst homeless people is probably that some of them fail to comply with treatment and then infect others with resistant organisms. Thus, in the Berne study described above, the homeless alcoholic subject thought to be the origin of the outbreak went on to develop a strain that was resistant first to isoniazid and then to rifampicin.[43] Similarly, in an outbreak that involved 60 people in Boston hostels for the homeless, the index case was a homeless person who had not been fully cured after initial diagnosis in 1968 owing to non-compliance with therapy.[49]

It is not clear how many homeless people who begin treatment for tuberculosis fail to complete the course, but small-scale studies give cause for concern. For example, one London study reported that one year after diagnosis only about a third of identified cases of active tuberculosis had been cured, failure being due largely to poor compliance.[44]

A considerable period may elapse before drug resistance is recognised, with the result that the homeless person sometimes receives inappropriate therapy and remains infectious for longer than is necessary.

Musculoskeletal disorders

Musculoskeletal disorders are common among homeless people, presumably as a result of trauma. Foot problems are particularly common. It has been claimed that up to 20% of the medical complaints of single homeless people are related to their feet.[60] There are four contributing factors. First, many homeless people do not lie down to sleep, and tend to keep their shoes on all the time to prevent them being stolen. The consequent blood pooling leads to chronic oedema and damage to the skin in the lower limbs, inflammation, infection and ulceration.[61] Second, standing or walking for long periods in ill-fitting or worn-out shoes, results in repetitive minor trauma to the feet. Third, alcoholism and poor nutrition lead to peripheral neuropathy and reduced pain sensation in the feet. Fourth, sleeping in wet footwear leads to 'trench foot', with secondary complications of infection, cellulitis and gangrene. Complications such as osteomyelitis and pyarthrosis occur in 3–10% of wound sites.[60]

Dermatological disorders, including infestations

The risk of infestation is increased by dirty clothes, lack of access to sanitary facilities, and exposure to infection in communal dwellings. Severe mental illness or substance dependence may also contribute by undermining motivation to maintain personal hygiene. Once established, infestations may prove difficult to treat because of lack of access to medical care or poor compliance.

Gastrointestinal problems, including disorders of the liver

There is fair agreement that gastrointestinal disorders are over-represented amongst homeless people in the UK, but little agreement as to the particular disorders. Surprisingly, given the high prevalence of alcohol abuse, there is little agreement that disorders of the liver are over-represented. It has been suggested that cirrhosis is uncommon amongst homeless alcoholics because they tend to drink intermittently, in binges when money is available,[51] so there are periods for the liver to recover.[12]

Neurological disorders and seizures

Neurological disorders, particularly epilepsy, are over-represented amongst homeless people. Chronic organic disorders such as dementia (due to progressive disorders such as Alzheimer's disease, or discrete cerebral insults such as head injury) may lead to a deterioration in social functioning that leads to homelessness by means similar to those described for schizophrenia (see Chapter 5). Homeless people are also prone to accidents or assaults that may result in permanent brain injury, as may excessive alcohol consumption or consumption of methylated spirits.

The high incidence of epilepsy amongst homeless people may be due to a number of reasons. First, epilepsy can be associated with factors that lead to homelessness, such as poor educational achievement and employment opportunities and impaired social functioning. Second, epilepsy is associated with other disorders that may lead to homelessness, such as head injury or mental retardation. Third, epilepsy may be a side-effect of drugs used for other disorders that are common amongst homeless people (such as schizophrenia). Fourth, epilepsy may be associated with alcohol dependence.

HIV infection

HIV infection among single homeless people is now recognised as a

major public health problem in the US. In New York, 9–18% of HIV
patients in hospitals are homeless, and between 5,000 and 8,000 of
the estimated 35,000–90,000 single homeless people in the city have
AIDS.[54] Homeless young people, amongst whom drug abuse, prostitution and sexually transmitted diseases are particularly common,[26]
are at particular risk of contracting HIV. It has been estimated that
about 4% of homeless youths in the US are HIV-positive, but the
figure increases to about 25% in populations where trading sex for
drugs or cash is a way of life. Approximately 50% of homeless youths
have had more than 10 sexual partners compared with only 7%
among the housed population. The rates of HIV infection amongst
homeless adults and young people in the UK are at present
unknown.

ALCOHOL AND SUBSTANCE ABUSE DISORDERS

Alcohol abuse prevalence studies

Data from the UK

In the UK there have been no recent studies of alcohol dependence
in single homeless people that are as comprehensive and systematic
as the American studies to be described later. Available studies are
summarised in Table 4.5. Surveys of attenders at Oxford GP clinics
for homeless people have shown that 60% of consultations are
for alcohol-related problems.[33] In Manchester, self-described
'alcoholism' accounted for 48% of consultations,[11] and 36% in
London were for alcohol abuse problems.[13] Among shelter populations, 61% of attenders at the Crisis at Christmas medical centre in
London reported self-diagnosed alcohol problems,[15] and 53% of
attenders at a London cold weather shelter showed alcohol dependence, as diagnosed by the Michigan Alcohol Screening Test
(MAST).[62] In a city-wide one-day census of single homeless people
in Sheffield, 28% of respondents described themselves as suffering
from 'alcoholism'.[8] Of the rough sleepers who consulted a mobile
surgery for the homeless in London, 47% were consuming more
than 56 units of alcohol per week.[18]

Data from the US

The American HCH program found that 38% of single homeless
people attending primary care clinics (47% males, 16% females)
were alcohol dependent.[1] Levels of alcohol dependence were found

TABLE 4.5   **Substance abuse in samples of the single (Group II) homeless, UK studies**

Study	Alcohol dependent (%)	Alcohol problem (%)	Drug problem (%)
Braddick	NR	61	NR
George	NR	28	9
Reed	27	53	37
Edwards	25	45	NR
Timms*	14	NR	1.5
Balazs	NR	49.3	13.5
Bines[a]	NR	13	3
[b]	NR	33	7
[c]	NR	30	9

NR = not reported.
[a]Hostel and B & B survey.
[b]Day Centre survey.
[c]Soup-run survey.
*New admissions.

to increase with age, from 22% in those aged under 30 years to 43% in those aged 50–65. In a sample of single homeless people in Baltimore, 85% of the men and 67% of the women were either current or previous abusers of alcohol.[23] In the same study the short form of MAST showed that 69% of men and 38% of women were currently dependent on alcohol.

Fischer[63] has estimated that alcohol dependence is nine times more common in single homeless people than in the general US population, probably because alcoholism leads to homelessness. This view is supported by a survey of homeless people in Los Angeles in which 80% said they lost their housing because of alcoholism.[64]

Drug abuse

Data from the UK

The extent of drug abuse in the UK homeless population is not clear, although we may assume that it is more widespread amongst young homeless people. Two broad patterns of abuse may be discerned: abuse of medication obtained from doctors and abuse of street drugs.

Within the former group, the most common category appears to be tranquilliser abuse. The HHELP project in east London has reported that approximately 10% of patients abuse minor tranquillisers (benzodiazepines or chlormethiazole), and most of these patients also abuse alcohol. This 'mixed dependency' causes particular problems for detoxification, as withdrawal periods may last for several weeks. Unintentional drug and alcohol overdoses are also reported by the HHELP team as a common cause of death.[12]

In a study in Sheffield, 9% (31 out of 340) of single homeless people surveyed claimed to abuse street drugs,[8] and 38% (37 out of 96) of people attending a cold weather shelter in London reported having used illicit drugs.[62] According to statistics gathered by the HHELP team, the commonest street drugs abused are cannabis (6.7% of all patients seen by the team), amphetamines (5.7%), cocaine (2.2%), opiates (1.4%) and LSD (1.1%).[12] Bines[9] found reported rates of dependency on non-prescribed drugs of 3% among hostel and B&B dwellers, 7% in day-centre users and 9% in soup-run users; the day-centre and soup-run users are rough sleepers.

Data from the US

The HCH program estimated that 13% of single homeless people were drug abusers.[1] Drug abuse was particularly common in the younger age groups. In Baltimore, 22% of men and 16% of women from a sample of homeless people were found to be drug dependent.[23] The incidence of intravenous drug abuse was twice as high among the homeless as in the housed people who attended a Californian free clinic, though neither rate was compared with national averages.[32]

Surveys in a number of North American cities have shown the extent of drug abuse among young homeless people. In Toronto, 41% of the street youth interviewed had injected drugs at least once in their lifetime, and 11% had shared needles during the previous year. A similar study in Hollywood (Los Angeles) found that 33% were drug abusers or drug dependent. It has been estimated that drug dependence is about five times greater among the street youth than in the housed population of the same age.[26]

ASPIRATIONS OF SINGLE HOMELESS PEOPLE

In the Department of the Environment report *Single homeless people*, Chapter 7 is entitled 'Accommodation expectations and preferences'.[65] The authors state:

'Despite the uncertain nature of respondents' current circumstances, the survey revealed a striking degree of consistency among single homeless people in their desire to obtain a home of their own, in which most felt they could manage with a modest level of support.'

Table 4.6 shows the preferred accommodation of the three samples and Table 4.7 shows the respondents' expressed needs for support in their preferred accommodation.

TABLE 4.6   **A survey of single homeless people showing their preferred accommodation**

| Preferred accommodation | Present accommodation/support | | |
	Hostel and B&B (%)	Day centre (%)	Soup run (%)
This accommodation	9	3	—
Own home	83	82	80
Parents' home	*	1	2
Friends'/relatives' home	*	*	—
Accommodation with job	1	2	3
Lodgings	1	1	2
Bed and breakfast hotel	*	1	3
Hostel/Resettlement unit	2	2	2
Old people's home/ sheltered housing	1	*	—
Sleeping rough/skippering	*	4	3
Other	1	2	3
No preference	*	1	*
Don't know/Couldn't respond	2	1	1
Total	*100*	*100*	*100*
Base	1,280	351	156

Base: All respondents.
Source: Department of the Environment, *Single homeless people.* London: HMSO, 1993. (Ref 65)
* Less than 1%.

Over 80% of respondents claimed that they would like their own home. About 60% recognised that they would need some support in such accommodation, including housekeeping, money management and social work help. Between 18% and 27% of respondents felt they would need medical support (Table 4.7).

TABLE 4.7   **Expressed needs of single homeless people for support in their preferred accommodation**

Support required	Present accommodation/support		
	Hostel and and B & B (% Yes)*	Day centre (% Yes)*	Soup run (% Yes)*
Housekeeping/ money management	27	32	35
Companionship	27	23	30
Medical help	18	19	27
Advice	37	33	43
Social work help	25	30	31
Other	6	6	3
At least one 'Yes'	*60*	*62*	*63*
Base	1,139	320	149

Base: All respondents who preferred some accommodation other than their current accommodation (see Table 4.6).
*Percentages do not sum to 100% as more than one answer could be given.
Source: Department of the Environment, *Single homeless people.* London: HMSO, 1993. (Ref 65)

References to Chapter 4 appear on page 129.

5 Mental health and homelessness

SUMMARY

- Serious mental illness is more common among single homeless people than in the general population.

- Schizophrenia is the most frequently observed serious disorder.

- Less serious disorders are also common amongst single homeless people.

- Factors associated with schizophrenia, combined with social and economic difficulties, increase the chance of a housing crisis which precipitates homelessness.

- Housing crises occur when there is inadequate integration of housing provision with social and health care as part of community care programmes.

- Housing policies must be reviewed and integrated with community care policies.

INTRODUCTION

This chapter first considers the evidence regarding the extent of mental disorder among single homeless people (Group II) and then describes how homelessness can arise from an interaction between social factors and symptoms produced by a major mental disorder. The example used is schizophrenia because it is the commonest major mental disorder among single homeless people and its prevalence is very much higher among them than in the general population.

PREVALENCE OF PSYCHIATRIC DISORDER AMONG SINGLE HOMELESS PEOPLE

Definition of mental disorder

A number of complex classifications of homeless people with mental illness have been proposed,[1] but simpler classifications will serve our purpose here. In this discussion mental disorders will be divided into two main groups: major mental disorders and neurotic disorders. These are defined as follows:

Major mental disorders are those that are likely to cause severe impairment of social functioning. The most common are schizophrenia and organic brain disease, but this category also includes severe depression and mania. At any one time, no more than 1% of the general population, under 70 years of age, is suffering from a major mental disorder. Before the arrival of community care most of those people severely affected by schizophrenia would have been long-stay patients.

Neurotic disorders include mild to moderate depression, anxiety disorders and adjustment disorders. These cause only mild impairment of social functioning and even before the advent of community care would not usually have led to long-term hospital treatment. The point prevalence of neurotic disorders in the general population is about 10%.

Review of prevalence studies in particular settings

Street dwellers

People who sleep exclusively on the streets and do not use hostels or shelters are difficult to study, but anecdotal evidence suggests that major mental disorder is very common among them.[2] Bines[3] also found that self-reported problems of 'depression, anxiety and nerves' were reported by 37% of rough sleepers using a day centre and by 41% of those using a soup run. These rates were about 10 times higher than those in a housed comparison group.

Night shelter users

Table 5.1 summarises the findings of prevalence studies conducted by psychiatrically trained interviewers of samples of people using

TABLE 5.1   **Prevalence of mental disorder amongst Group II homeless surveyed in night shelters***

Study	Year	All major mental disorder (%)	Schizophrenia (%)	Previous psychiatric admission (%)
Tidmarsh	1970	16	NR	29
Timms (new arrivals)	1989	26.5	25	NR
George	1991	NR	NR	32.19
Reed	1992	12	NR	18

NR = not reported.
*One night stays.

British shelters and reception centres. The studies indicate a prevalence of major mental disorder ranging from 12% to 26.5% (mean 18.2%).[4-7] There is insufficient evidence to determine how far the major mental disorder in question is schizophrenia. The prevalence of neurotic disorders in the users of shelters and reception centres is unknown.

Hostel dwellers

Studies in large hostels and the now largely defunct common lodging houses have consistently reported very high levels of major mental disorder, with schizophrenia by far the most common (Table 5.2). All the studies except that of Geddes indicate a prevalence of

TABLE 5.2   **Prevalence of mental disorder in UK studies of hostel populations**

Study	Year of publication	Major mental disorder (%)	Schizophrenia (%)
Tidmarsh	1970	29[a]	NR
Lodge-Patch	1971	18	15
Priest	1976	32	26
Timms (residents)	1989	39	37
Marshall M	1989	32.88	27.4
Marshall EJ	1992	68.57	64.29
Adams	1993	NR	50
Geddes	1994	NR	9

[a]Includes mental handicap and affective disorders.
NR = not reported.

major mental disorder ranging from 18% to 68.5%.[4,5,8-13] The prevalence of schizophrenia ranges from 9% to 64%. The highest prevalence of major mental disorder appears to be found in more recent studies and in hostels for homeless women.[11,12]

There is evidence to suggest that the mentally ill people found in hostels are often severely socially disabled and have many unmet social, psychiatric and medical needs.[10,14]

There is some disagreement over the extent of neurotic disorders in hostel users.[15] Evidence from American epidemiological studies suggests that neurotic disorder is present in approximately 45% of single homeless men and 70% of single homeless women,[16] but caution must be exercised in extrapolating from American to British homeless populations. Neurotic symptoms are certainly common.[10] Studies of UK resettlement units have reported high levels of distress on the General Health Questionnaire in 30–50% of residents,[17] but in many cases these symptoms of neurotic disorder may coexist with major mental disorder. In a secondary analysis of the 1991 representative sample survey of single homeless people, 27% of hostel and B&B dwellers complained of 'depression, anxiety or nerves'.[3] When compared with the general population, this sample had a standardised morbidity ratio for 'depression, anxiety or nerves' of 789 (standard population = 100).

Poor quality bedsits

There are anecdotal reports that considerable numbers of mentally ill people live in extremely poor quality accommodation in the private sector — in bedsits and other multiple occupancy houses. Data are not available on the extent of this phenomenon.

Has the number of homeless mentally ill people increased in recent years?

Most commentators agree that the number of homeless mentally ill people has increased in recent years.[1,18-22] Surprisingly, there is only a limited amount of relevant empirical evidence to support this view, but there is only one study that contradicts it.[13]

(i) Data from GP clinics for homeless people and from hostels

An increasing number of GP clinics for homeless people have been established in recent years and these have tended to report an increase in the number of patients seen, including those with mental disorders. For example, data from a GP clinic for homeless people in Oxford reported a 250% increase both in the total number of patients seen during 1981–9 and in the number with mental illness.[23] Whilst this finding is consistent with an increase in the number of homeless mentally ill people in Oxford, there are a number of other plausible explanations for it, not least the tendency of a service to attract more clients as it matures.

Hostels for homeless people have also reported an increase in the number of homeless mentally ill people requesting admission.[24] In 1989, the St Mungo's community in London reported a five-fold increase in the number of homeless mentally ill people seeking a bed for the night in its London hostels. The community reported that half of those seeking a hostel bed were now mentally disordered.[25]

(ii) Comparison of current prevalence studies with earlier studies

It might be possible to determine whether there has been an increase in the number of homeless people with mental disorders by comparing earlier prevalence rates for mental disorder with data from more recent studies. Unfortunately there are few suitable data from before 1959, when a Royal Commission on mental illness and mental disorder first recommended a shift to care in the community. The best available data are from a 1956 study of 19 Glasgow common lodging houses which found that only 19 (2.3%) of 800 residents were suffering from schizophrenia.[26] A study of Edinburgh common lodging houses in 1966 indicated that 26% of residents had schizophrenia.[9] A follow-up study of Edinburgh hostels for homeless people reported a prevalence of only 9%.[13] The authors conclude that their findings 'are not consistent with an increase in the prevalence of schizophrenia among homeless people, despite a 66% reduction in adult psychiatric beds in the region during 1966–92.' However, the sampling frames and case definitions in the 1992 study were different from those in the earlier study and there were high levels of non-response (31%). Although the authors attempted to adjust for possible confounding by age and current hostel use, these factors may have resulted in systematic bias (for example, some hostels are less likely than others to accept mentally ill residents). Therefore, it is not clear how far this study shows a decrease in the prevalence of schizophrenia among hostel residents.[27] Studies of the prevalence of mental illness in UK hostels are summarised in Table 5.2. Overall they suggest that in recent years hostels have catered for increasing numbers of mentally disordered people. Although numerous methodological difficulties preclude any firm conclusions being drawn, the existence of significant numbers of seriously mentally ill people in night shelters and in hostels indicates that appropriate housing must be better integrated into community care planning, implementation and monitoring. This is discussed further in Chapter 6. One possible solution to the problems of caring for patients who are difficult to place, or who comply poorly with medication, is to link the payment of benefits to the receipt of treatment. For example, within assertive community treatment programs in the US, it is common practice to pay patients' benefits directly to their key worker or case manager through 'protective payee accounts.'[28] This form of payment enables case managers to determine, for example, where patients live, and presumably to reward them financially for compliant behaviour. The disadvantage of this approach is that it is out of keeping with the frequently expressed value of 'empowering' patients,[29] and would not be in keeping with the Government's present policy on community care. Whilst the 'protective payee' approach might have advantages for some patients, its introduction in the UK could not be recommended without very careful consideration of its effectiveness, and the curtailment of civil rights that it entails.

SCHIZOPHRENIA AND HOMELESSNESS

Two explanations have been put forward for the association between schizophrenia and homelessness, neither of which is entirely satisfactory. The first is that the high prevalence of schizophrenia among homeless people is due to the closure of large mental institutions,[30] since an upsurge in the number of homeless mentally ill people has accompanied the closure of asylums both in the UK and in the US. There may be a connection between hospital closures, a decrease in the number of inpatient beds and the increase in the number of homeless mentally ill people, but research suggests that this is not a simple cause and effect relationship. Studies of the closure of long-stay hospitals and the community placement of long-stay patients have shown that only very small numbers of such patients become homeless. Moreover, contemporary studies of homeless mentally ill people suggest that, whilst many have had brief admissions to hospital, few have been long-stay patients.[31]*

---

*In this research, 'long-stay' has various definitions. In general it is used to describe people who have been inpatients for five years or more. People who have been inpatients for two to five years are described as 'new long-stay'.

The second explanation for the high prevalence of schizophrenia among single homeless people is that homelessness is such a traumatic experience that it causes schizophrenia.[21] This hypothesis may seem plausible, but there is little evidence to support it, and three major arguments against it. First, reports of the onset of schizophrenia following homelessness are exceptional, whilst reports of people with schizophrenia becoming homeless are very common.[23,32,33] Second, schizophrenia is a relatively uncommon condition. Although adverse life events, such as homelessness, double the relative risk of developing schizophrenia over the subsequent six months,[34] this does not nearly account for the fact that this disorder is fifty to a hundred times more common in single homeless people than in the general population. Third, members of homeless families have also experienced many threatening life events, but they do not show excess rates of schizophrenia.[35]

It is therefore not likely that the stress of homelessness explains the association with schizophrenia.

Reasons for homelessness amongst people with schizophrenia

The actual relationship between schizophrenia and homelessness is complex and involves the interplay of features of the disorder and social factors.

Features of schizophrenia that contribute to homelessness

Five features of schizophrenia may contribute to sufferers becoming homeless:

1 *Impairment of life skills*

People severely affected by schizophrenia (about one-third of the total population with the disorder) lack social skills and have low levels of social competence.[36,37] They tend to be socially withdrawn, poorly motivated and frequently lack basic life skills such as washing and dressing, communicating effectively, planning ahead, managing money and using public transport. As a result they suffer social handicaps and tend to be poor, unemployed, unmarried, isolated and hence prone to homelessness.[38] A recent study of hostels for the homeless in Oxford found that one in three residents (48 out of 152) were socially disabled by mental illness. Half of these were as disabled as the most severely affected long-stay hospital patients, and 40 of them had a diagnosis of schizophrenia.[10]

2 *Socially unacceptable behaviour*

Some people with schizophrenia display socially unacceptable behaviour which can be threatening, bizarre or sexually offensive. Such behaviour is not well tolerated by members of the public and may lead to loss of accommodation.

3 *Fluctuating course*

People with schizophrenia who are normally free of symptoms may relapse, and those who are already socially disabled may suffer exacerbations of the disease. A common consequence of such relapses or exacerbations is that established living arrangements can no longer be sustained. A study of short-stay admissions to a London psychiatric hospital showed that 40% of inpatients lost their accommodation during the admission.[39]

4 *Secondary problems*

Some people with schizophrenia may also develop secondary problems such as substance abuse or depression that make it difficult for them to keep their accommodation. Substance abuse is one way of attempting to relieve the symptoms of schizophrenia, but it generally leads to further deterioration, reduction in social competence and aggravation of socially unacceptable behaviour. It is therefore a major impediment to keeping accommodation,[7] and there is evidence that coexisting diagnoses of schizophrenia and substance abuse are common among homeless mentally ill people.[1]

Depression is common in schizophrenia and can affect social competence by further reducing motivation and energy. Depressive symptoms also appear to be common amongst homeless people with schizophrenia.[10]

5 *Insight*

People with schizophrenia commonly lack insight into the nature of their disorder.[40] Despite repeated relapses they may not see the value of medication. They may adhere to unrealistic beliefs about their social situation and may view with suspicion efforts to assist them. The persistent failure of such people to comply with medication and follow-up can sometimes make it impossible to avoid homelessness, even when well developed community services are available.

Social factors that contribute to homelessness amongst people with schizophrenia

General factors

Both the shortage of low-cost housing in the social-rented and private-rented sectors and the increasingly competitive job market contribute to the general problem of homelessness (Chapters 1 and 2). People with schizophrenia are particularly affected by these factors because they suffer from social disabilities that put them at a disadvantage when competing for accommodation and employment.

Specific factors

People with schizophrenia are at particular risk of homelessness because of:

Lack of social support — People with schizophrenia tend to remain single, lose contact with their families, and have few friends,[29] so at times of crisis they often have no one to turn to for assistance.

Changes in the provision of psychiatric care — Certain deficiencies in the provision of psychiatric care have increased the risk of homelessness for people with schizophrenia. There has been a failure to provide suitable accommodation for new chronically ill patients.[41] Community support for such patients has been inadequate, because of a shortage of community psychiatric nurses working with them, bureaucratic barriers that prevent patients from receiving prompt assistance, failure to follow up patients who do not attend appointments, concentration of resources on the less severely ill, and disagreement about responsibility for difficult patients. The increasing emphasis on patient autonomy within the mental health professions and in mental health legislation has meant that mental health workers are unwilling or unable to deflect some patients from action that will make homelessness inevitable.[32] It is too early to evaluate the impact of the CARE Programme Approach, care management and other recent legislation, such as supervision registers, in combating this unsatisfactory state of affairs.

Discrimination against people with mental disorders — People with schizophrenia tend to be housed in the worst accommodation in the most dilapidated inner-city areas, out of choice or through financial necessity or because these are the areas where mentally ill people are best tolerated.[42] Attempts to open group homes in better residential areas have sometimes resulted in legal proceedings.[43] Whilst it is difficult to determine how far adverse public attitudes contribute to homelessness among people with mental illness, these attitudes exist and their potential effects should not be discounted.

How social factors interact with features of schizophrenia to cause homelessness

The model described below is helpful in describing the relationships between social and illness factors that can cause homelessness in people with schizophrenia. It uses the term 'housing crisis' which is defined as a situation that demands immediate action if one is to retain accommodation or find new accommodation and so avoid homelessness. The model is based on clinical experience, supported by research evidence where available.

1 *Factors that predispose to a housing crisis*

People who suffer from schizophrenia are likely to be unemployed and to have low incomes. In the absence of supported or subsidised accommodation they gravitate towards cheap, poor quality housing at the bottom end of the privately rented sector and may even be placed there by the psychiatric services, because suitable supported accommodation is unavailable. This type of poor quality accommodation is inherently insecure and in increasingly short supply, so residents live at risk of a housing crisis.

2 *Factors that precipitate a housing crisis*

Often a housing crisis will be precipitated by extraneous factors such as unscrupulous landlords, urban renewal or price rises. A housing crisis can also occur as a result of a relapse or exacerbation of the disorder, failure to comply with medication or an episode of socially unacceptable behaviour. At such times hospital admission may be an opportunity for landlords to dispose of awkward or embarrassing tenants. Finally, a housing crisis may arise simply through failure to pay bills, because of disorganisation and lack of forward planning, due to substance abuse or because of poverty.

3 *Factors that prevent a housing crisis from being resolved*

People with schizophrenia are poorly equipped to cope with a housing crisis. Their disease results in a lack of motivation, lack of financial resources and inadequate social skills. These factors combine in many cases with lack of support from friends and family.

When inpatient beds are in short supply and community psychiatric services are poor or overstretched, as is often the case in deprived areas, there may be no one to turn to for assistance. So, for many, a housing crisis ends in homelessness.[44]

4 *Factors that maintain homelessness*

Once people with schizophrenia become 'roofless' their chances of being rehoused are poor. Without an address, they are likely to lose all contact with the psychiatric and social services, resulting in failure to take medication and further deterioration. Some become rough sleepers, but in the UK the majority of homeless people with schizophrenia probably find their way to hostels for the homeless.

Hostels provide shelter and a degree of support, but they themselves are not well supported by the statutory services, so their residents may have many unmet medical, psychiatric and social needs.[14] There are case reports of people with schizophrenia remaining in hostels for years without suitable medical treatment which, when finally provided, greatly improved their condition.[45] Such lack of professional care, sometimes justified on the basis of 'autonomy', allows further deterioration, makes resettlement impossible and means that residents suffering from mental illness tend to remain in hostels longer than other residents.[5,10]

Even when hostel residents are suitable for resettlement it appears that they do not fare well in obtaining suitable supported accommodation. A follow-up of 48 mentally ill residents of Oxford hostels found that none of the 10 who were rehoused after 18 months was placed in accommodation supported by the psychiatric or social services.[23] The problems of these residents appear to be compounded by the addition of the stigma of homelessness to that of mental illness.

MENTAL DISORDER, HOMELESSNESS AND THE CRIMINAL JUSTICE SYSTEM

High levels of criminal activity and high levels of arrests and previous imprisonment are consistently reported among single homeless people.[1] A survey of residents of a cold weather shelter in London found that 71% had previous convictions and 52% had served custodial sentences,[7] whilst a census of single homeless people in Sheffield found that 152 out of 292 men (52%) had been imprisoned.[6]

Rates of imprisonment and arrest are also high among mentally disordered homeless people. An Oxford study of hostel residents suffering from severe mental disorder found that 48% had served custodial sentences and 27% had been arrested during the previous 12 months.[10] Mentally disordered homeless people are more likely to be imprisoned than those who have no mental disorder,[17] and they are commonly arrested for minor offences. Of 334 men remanded to Winchester prison for psychiatric reports, 59% were homeless on arrest and most had committed only minor offences.[46] The findings of this study were supported by a study of the duty psychiatry scheme at Horseferry Road magistrate's court which found that two-thirds of the 80 people referred were homeless.[47]

Among the prison population itself mental illness is also common.[48] A recent random survey based on a 5% sample of men in 16 prisons found that 652 out of 1,365 men (47%) had psychiatric disorders, and 49 were suffering from psychosis or organic disorders. By extrapolation it was estimated that the sentenced prison population contained over 700 men with psychosis and around 1,100 who would warrant transfer to hospital for psychiatric treatment. Many of these people are at risk of homelessness following discharge from prison. These findings emphasise the need for an expansion of court diversion schemes.[47]

RECOMMENDATION 6

Within the wide-ranging policy review (see Chapter 2, Recommendation 2)

i Community care of severely mentally ill people requires full implementation of the Care Programme Approach and care management. Both should explicitly include adequate housing as an essential component. Community care should be seen as a combination of appropriate care and appropriate housing.

ii Community care plans drawn up by local authorities and health authorities should specify the housing requirements of severely mentally ill people. Central government should ensure that resources are available for capital developments (buildings and renovation), rehabilitation and support.

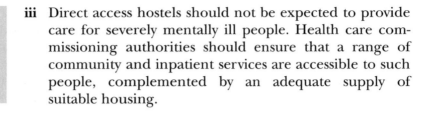

iii Direct access hostels should not be expected to provide care for severely mentally ill people. Health care commissioning authorities should ensure that a range of community and inpatient services are accessible to such people, complemented by an adequate supply of suitable housing.

References to Chapter 5 appear on page 133.

6 Services for homeless people

SUMMARY

- Homeless people experience difficulties in obtaining health care.
- The mobility of homeless families may leave them at a distance from their own primary care services.
- Single homeless people may be unable or unwilling to use normal services and may have difficulty in registering with a GP.
- Many homeless people leave hospital with inadequate post-discharge arrangements.
- The NHS reforms may adversely affect the care of homeless people.
- Proposed changes in homelessness legislation may further hinder access to care.
- Special arrangements for homeless people are needed for:
  - primary care
  - A&E services
  - discharge plans
  - community care.

INTRODUCTION

We have distinguished in this report three groups of homeless people who have different health needs and face different barriers in obtaining access to health care and other welfare services. Although they are likely to exist, the health problems and health care needs specific to Group III homeless people (those in insecure accommodation) have not been researched and described in any useful detail. This chapter therefore considers only the constraints to access and delivery of health care for Group I and Group II

91

homeless people, and comments, where appropriate, on health care and housing policy. The emphasis is on services managed by the NHS, although effective collaboration with non-NHS agencies is of central importance.

CONSTRAINTS AND BARRIERS TO ACCESS

Group I homeless people

These are typically couples with children of pre-school age, single mothers and pregnant women who have been placed in temporary accommodation such as B&B hotels and private sector leased accommodation. Their characteristics and health problems are described in Chapters 1 and 3.

Many homeless families are placed in temporary accommodation far from their GP, and many are moved involuntarily several times before being permanently housed, making registration with a new GP impractical. In this situation many opt for temporary registration, which hinders continuity of care because medical records are not transferred. Understandably, many do not bother to register with a new GP and so have to travel substantial distances or use A&E departments to receive care.

This mobility also causes problems for care providers. Health visitors are often not notified when a homeless family is moved into their area, and must rely on hotel managers or existing clients to inform them. The health visitors may not have access to medical records and therefore may not know the children's immunisation history. These problems are compounded in places where there is a large ethnic minority population with associated language problems. Similar difficulties are experienced by other agencies, for example by social services departments following up children on Child Protection registers who are considered to be at risk of abuse.

The NHS service development project Access to Health, set up by three Thames Regions, has identified the following services as being essential for homeless families:
  – GPs
  – Health visiting
  – Dentistry
  – Support/counselling
  – School nursing.

Access to a general practitioner is particularly important to ensure access and coordination of services. Improvements could also be achieved by greater flexibility, for example by allowing pregnant women to refer themselves to midwives when they do not have a GP, and allowing mothers with young children to hold their own health records.

The report *Prescription for Poor Health*[1] recommended higher staffing levels in community services in areas with many homeless families. A ratio of at least one health visitor per 50 families was suggested, with outreach services, such as antenatal and baby clinics, supported by interpreters and translated literature where needed.

Group II homeless people

Group II homeless people are those who sleep rough or use night shelters, direct access hostels and B&B hotels. They are described in detail in Chapter 1, and evidence of their health status is set out in Chapter 4.

This information would indicate that the health care needs of Group II homeless people are greater than those of the general population. However, within this group there are diverse health needs, related to age and environmental exposure. These factors need to be matched by diverse and flexible services. It is therefore important that the health needs of the local homeless population be properly assessed before embarking on the planning and delivery of services.

Local health services should take account of two aspects of the health needs of homeless people: their experience of existing services and the health-damaging effects of homelessness.[2]

Access to primary care

The GP is often referred to as the gatekeeper of the health service who '. . . controls the patients' access to . . . a range of health care resources, including prescribed drugs and medicines and most hospital and consultant services'.[3]

A person can receive treatment from a GP through three main arrangements—permanent registration, temporary registration and emergency treatment:

Permanent registration. Every person has a statutory right to register with a GP, but the GP is not obliged to accept a person requesting registration unless assigned to his/her list by the Family Health Services Authority (FHSA). A homeless person may be refused registration because of the lack of a permanent address (although some FHSAs are willing to accept the address of a day centre or hostel or the FHSA itself), or because the GP will accept only patients living within a given radius of the surgery, which excludes people who are of 'no fixed abode'. The problem of access appears to be particularly acute for rough sleepers since GPs may register hostel dwellers but not people living on the streets.

Some GPs have complained that the itinerant lifestyle of homeless people constitutes a financial and administrative disincentive to permanent registration. For example, if a GP registers a person who moves and registers elsewhere before the end of the quarter, the capitation fee is forfeited regardless of how much treatment that person has received during the period. The new GP contract also creates a disincentive to work with disadvantaged and mobile groups because they make health promotion targets more difficult to achieve.

Temporary registration (for 3 months or less) and *Emergency treatment.* These arrangements present less financial or administrative worry since medical records are not transferred from the previous GP and a capitation fee is received for the quarter. However, these forms of registration were designed chiefly for the treatment of visitors and people temporarily working away from home. They cannot provide the continuity of care that homeless people require.

Some GPs are reluctant to offer any form of registration to homeless people because of concern about their behaviour and its possible effect on other patients. A survey of GPs in Manchester in 1980 found that many GPs still expected a homeless person to be a 'dirty, drunken and abusive middle-aged male' who would be disruptive and unacceptable to other patients in the reception area.[4] Many felt that treating such a person would require more time and resources than are available. GPs are also concerned about the lack of social worker support for single homeless people and especially for drug and alcohol abusers.

GP reluctance cannot be the only explanation for poor access to primary care among single homeless people since registration among hostel dwellers is relatively high in some areas.[5,6] In east London, 70% of users of the HHELP project were registered with a GP,[5] as were 63% of single homeless people in West Lambeth.[7] These figures, however, conceal a wide disparity between hostel dwellers (83% registered) and rough sleepers (35% registered). Of those who were not registered, 82% had never attempted to do so, mainly because they expected to be refused. Others said GP registration was a lower priority than finding a bed for the night or getting a hot meal.

The reluctance of homeless people to use GP services, even if registered, coupled with the unwillingness of some GPs to accept them can result in what has been described as a 'cycle of reluctance.'[8] Personal or reported refusal of registration further diminishes the self-esteem of the homeless person who, in expectation of refusal, does not attempt to use GP services. Health may be given a low priority until an illness reaches crisis point. Low health expectation may also explain the postponement of health care until illness has become serious.[9] This theory suggests that the failure to seek help early in the course of disease is a rational decision by homeless people, who expect and accept that illness is inevitable in their situation.

Access to accident and emergency services

Given the difficulties of obtaining primary care, the open access and 24-hour availability of accident and emergency departments make them the most easily accessible source of health care for most homeless people. However, they are often perceived to be abusing the facility and seeking shelter rather than medical care, though there appears to be little evidence to support this view. The West Lambeth study reported that 75% of rough sleepers who had recently attended an A&E department did so because of injury or assault,[7] and a study in Manchester showed that 70.5% of the homeless people presenting at an A&E department were in genuine need of casualty treatment or immediate admission.

On the other hand, there is evidence that many of the presenting conditions would be more appropriately treated in primary care. For example, Powell found that the appropriateness of A&E consultations was as low as 29% among homeless people, compared with 75% in the general population.[10]

Discharge and aftercare

The rate of unplanned admissions to hospitals has been found to be high amongst all sections of the homeless population. Stern *et al*[7] estimated that homeless people in West Lambeth used inpatient services two and a half times as often as the general population, while Scheuer *et al*[11] estimated that homeless people in London were twice as likely to use acute services. Hostel dwellers were found to have a significantly longer average length of stay in hospital than people living in bed and breakfast or temporary leased accommodation (18 days vs 4 days or less). These figures suggest that homeless people are both frequent and intensive users of services. Readmission rates are also believed to be high among homeless people, which may be due to the current trend towards early discharge and to inadequate aftercare facilities. Failure to acknowledge the lack of family and friends has resulted in homeless people being discharged with advice such as 'go home, take bed rest and see your GP in the morning.'[12] The reality of discharge is often back onto the streets or into hostels or other temporary accommodation where the conditions are totally unsuitable for convalescence. It is likely that there will be no qualified staff and inappropriate building design with cramped living conditions, too many stairs and in-convenient toilets and bathing facilities. Many hostels do not provide meals or shelter during the day.[13]

Particular problems may be experienced in planning for the discharge of people who require treatment in alcohol detoxification units (see page 111). The combination of inappropriate discharge policies and the inadequate aftercare may be expected to result in a poor outcome of hospital treatment for homeless people.

HEALTH AND SOCIAL SERVICE PROVISION

We now discuss health and housing policy issues and developments, and attempt to identify a fair, coordinated and practical pattern of health and housing services, responsive to the needs of homeless people.

1 Primary care

Three main systems of primary health care for homeless people have been proposed.

Model A: A fully integrated service

This approach asserts that improved flexibility, co-ordination and co-operation within the existing health and social care institutions would allow homeless people to be fully integrated into mainstream services. Critics of this approach argue that while it is a commend-able idea it is also an impossible one to achieve under the current structure of primary and secondary health services and the current arrangements for the provision of social care; they also argue that this ideal cannot address the immediate health care needs of home-less people. It is, however, the most appropriate model for Group I homeless families.

Model B: Special schemes to improve access

These schemes provide clinics for homeless people in special premises, day centres or hostels, with a view to transferring care to mainstream services. A common problem of such projects is the 'mixed message' for the homeless person, who is encouraged to use the special service and build a relationship with a health professional who then tries to refer them to another service.[5] Furthermore, some schemes have found difficulty in identifying mainstream GPs who are willing to accept homeless people.

Model C: Separate services

This approach asserts that under the current structure of health services full integration of homeless people is unlikely in the foreseeable future and that their health care needs can only be met by special services which cater exclusively for them. Such services are typically provided within hostels and day centres or special walk-in clinics. It is argued that these services are preferred by homeless people, who would not feel comfortable in the often hostile environment of a normal GP surgery. However, critics argue that such services absolve GPs and others from their duty to treat homeless people and further perpetuate their isolation and stigmatisation. There is also concern that some groups of homeless people, particularly women, may be discouraged from attending clinics held in predominantly male hostels.

Some of the primary care services which are provided for Group II homeless people are described in Appendix A and examples of services for homeless families are described in Appendix B. Whilst none of the schemes conforms to the ideal of fully integrated provision, they illustrate the current responses of both statutory and voluntary organisations to the needs of homeless people.

2 Accident and emergency services

Until the necessary improvements in primary care occur, it is likely that A&E departments will continue to be used as a principal source of care by homeless people. It is essential therefore that they become better equipped to treat homeless people sensitively and effectively and are adequately resourced to provide such care.

Access to Health has outlined elements of good practice for the provision of NHS services to homeless people.[14] For A&E services they recommend:

• Appropriate training of staff in how to deal with homeless people in a sensitive and effective way.

- Availability of up-to-date information on resources available to homeless people in the community (eg hostels, soup kitchens, housing departments) and how to make referrals to them. This can be done by a non-medical homelessness worker/co-ordinator within the A&E department.
- The employment of GPs on a sessional basis, not only to ease the pressure on A&E departments but also to improve communication between primary care workers and hospitals.

3 Admission and discharge from acute services

It has been suggested that a liaison officer should be appointed within the Homeless Persons Unit of the relevant local authority to undertake outreach work. Such an officer would assess homeless people who are currently being treated for mental illness in hospitals or other institutions. This officer would collaborate with hospital staff and take the lead in assessing the housing needs of the patient, involving the relevant statutory and voluntary agencies in securing adequate accommodation and support before the individual is discharged. This arrangement would also be appropriate for homeless people receiving acute non-psychiatric care. The general requirements of good discharge policy and practice are especially pertinent in dealing with homeless people.[15] Successful implementation requires adequate professional and management resources and good collaboration between health authorities and local authority housing and social services departments.[16]

- Discharge of homeless people from all acute departments requires clear, coordinated policy. Staff should liaise with housing and social services departments and voluntary organisations to secure appropriate accommodation and convalescent care on discharge.

Examples of good practice in discharge arrangements are given in Appendix C.

4 Community care and homelessness

The failure of mainstream health care services to meet the needs of homeless people no doubt accounts for the proliferation of special services described in Appendices A and B, but it is also becoming apparent that newer policy initiatives such as the NHS and Community Care Act 1990 have similarly failed to recognise the needs of homeless people.[17] This Act and the guidance accompanying it sets out local authorities' responsibility to assess the needs of, and to provide care and support to, people who are vulnerable for reasons of health or age. Specific care groups identified in the policy are elderly people and those suffering from substance abuse and AIDS. All of these groups are represented in the homeless population, yet their homelessness is *de facto* evidence that they are falling through the community care net. Moreover, the guidance makes no mention of how this already underserved group gain access to care in the community. The barriers to health care described above apply in the same ways to community care.

In addition, a number of institutional barriers exist. Local authorities will only accept responsibility for people who can provide proof of 'ordinary residence' or of a local connection (eg family ties to the area). Furthermore, it is implicitly assumed that those entitled to a needs assessment will already be in contact with a GP or one of the statutory services. However, the reality is that many homeless people will have lost contact with such bodies, and may be receiving both care and accommodation through the voluntary sector, which therefore must be specifically integrated into the community care network.

5 Community care and mental illness

Care in the Community was explicitly targeted at mentally ill people. However, in the transition from institutional care to the community, many mentally ill people have found themselves placed in inappropriate settings in which they become isolated, lose contact with health and social services agencies and eventually become homeless. People suffering from mental illness may then find it particularly difficult to gain access to the network of community health, housing and social services.[17]

Inappropriate discharge of patients from short-stay and, perhaps less important, long-stay mental institutions has been implicated in the increasing number of people with mental disorders on the streets. The Care Programme Approach (CPA), which was introduced by the Department of Health in 1990, aimed to encourage a more systematic approach to patient discharge and to ensure that proper arrangements are made for continuing health and social care of patients in the community. It recommended that if minimum health and social care needs of patients could not be met in the community, they should continue to be offered inpatient treatment. There should be regular reviews of such treatment and of the resources available in the community. Each discharged patient should have a 'key worker' who is a named professional with responsibility for monitoring care and for informing health and social services departments of any relevant changes in the patient's circumstances.[18] The Health Committee of the House of Commons gathered extensive evidence which showed that there remain institutional, management, resource and professional barriers to the integration of housing and community care services for mentally ill people.[17] It recommended a thorough review of the existing un-coordinated policies.

6 Community care for people with problems of substance abuse or addiction

Concerns have been raised over the implications of the new Community Care financing arrangements for people needing care for substance abuse, since the cost of residential care is no longer met by the Department of Social Security. The funding has been transferred to local authorities, who may buy such care but may reject homeless people unless they have proof of a local connection. Furthermore, despite earlier assurance that funding for specialist drug and alcohol services would be safeguarded, the final legislation did not include ringfenced funding. Many of these services operate over wide geographical areas which are not coterminous with health or local authority boundaries. Many local authorities are unwilling to fund projects that also serve people from other areas and, since they have no statutory responsibility to provide drug and alcohol services, these services are unlikely to appear high on any list of priorities.[19]

7 The provision of housing under community care

Intuitively one would expect the provision of stable accommodation to have two principal effects on the health of homeless people. It would improve health status, because of reduced risk of illnesses associated with street or hostel living. It would also improve access to health care through removal of the barriers created by the lack of a permanent address.

The provision of housing and the provision of social support are closely bound together. We support the view that housing should be redefined as a basic requirement of community care,[20-22] but housing has been given only minor consideration in legislation, official guidelines and local authority community care plans.[17,22] In spite of a circular issued jointly by the Department of Health and the Department of the Environment emphasising the need for housing authorities to cooperate fully in planning and assessment processes,[23] a recent review of the community care plans of ten districts found that housing departments were not adequately involved, and the plans tended to be dominated by health and social services authorities.[21] Cooperation is poor even in areas where housing and social services departments lie within the same authority. It is further complicated by logistical problems in counties where one social service department may find itself coterminous with several district housing authorities, each with its own housing policy.[24] Examples of good joint practice are set out in Appendix D.

8 Vulnerability

The definitions of vulnerability under the 1985 Housing Act are open to discretionary interpretation by local authorities, and the stringency of eligibility criteria is often determined by the supply of available housing. People seeking housing on the grounds of medical need or vulnerability often face a lengthy process which can be daunting, particularly for those with chronic physical or mental illness. Applicants are often expected to produce documentary medical evidence from their GPs which can be difficult for homeless people who are not registered. Moreover, as Smith points out, the Medical Priority for Rehousing (MPR) system offers homeless people *less* not more opportunity than non-homeless MPR applicants.[25]

It is clear that, owing to the current growing demand for local authority and housing association housing and the limited supply, single homeless people remain low on housing priority lists. Inconsistencies in eligibility criteria are such that it is possible for a homeless mentally ill person to fail to meet the criteria of the housing department even when assessed as vulnerable by social services. Harmonisation of housing and social services procedures and eligibility criteria would greatly improve the situation.[25]

The provision of suitable housing is also a key part of the discharge arrangements for homeless patients or those leaving psychiatric care.[17]

It has been suggested that the interpretation of vulnerability be widened to include:

• single homeless people forced to sleep rough;
• young homeless people who would be considered in need under the Children Act;

- homeless people with drug or alcohol problems.[26]

These groups should be given emergency temporary accommodation with a view to further assessment and placement in suitable long-term settings.

9 Potential effects of the NHS reforms on the health care of homeless people

It is difficult at this stage to predict accurately the effect of the NHS reforms on health care for homeless people. However, some effects seem likely:

The reforms will make GPs less willing to register homeless people

GPs may be unwilling to accept homeless patients because:

- GPs now receive payments for the achievement of health targets. If a GP registers large numbers of homeless people, it is less likely that he or she will achieve these targets, and hence will face financial penalties.
- Homeless people are unattractive to GP fundholders because they have high levels of morbidity and hence will consume more of the fundholder's budget than the average housed patient. In addition, financially attractive housed patients may be reluctant to share practice facilities with disadvantaged homeless people, who may be mentally ill or have drug and alcohol problems. If the housed patients exercise their right to switch to practices that do not register homeless patients, the practices that do cater for homeless people will be at a financial disadvantage.

The reforms will make it more difficult for homeless people to obtain non-urgent care

Homeless people are more likely than housed people to cross the boundaries of district health authorities. Having done so, they are likely to encounter problems registering with local GPs. If they then require elective treatment, a hospital Trust or unit may refuse to provide this treatment without a guarantee of payment from the health authority in which the patient was originally registered, which may be unwilling to sanction expenditure on someone with only tenuous links with the district. At best this is likely to lead to delays in obtaining hospital treatment for homeless people; at worst it may lead to treatment being refused altogether.

The reforms will reduce the effectiveness of special practices currently providing primary care to homeless people

At present much primary health care for homeless people is provided by one of four types of special practice:

• Practices directly funded by central government, usually as pilot projects.

• Small branch surgeries which are part of existing GP practices and depend largely on donations and fees for temporary registration.

• Services provided on a sessional basis at hostels by arrangement with local GPs who run clinics at fixed times for fixed fees.

• Services provided gratis by sympathetic GPs.

Under the NHS reforms, these special practices will be unable to obtain care for their patients as effectively as fundholding practices because they cannot hold their own budgets and hence cannot pay for treatment, so their patients who require elective care are likely to be given a low priority by hospital Trusts. These special practices have a greater need to buy care than fundholding practices, because of the poor health of their homeless patients, but will have less money available per patient.

Inconsistencies in allocations to District Health Authorities

At present, Regional Health Authorities (NHS Executive Regional Offices after 1996) decide on formulae for the distribution of funds to purchasing authorities. These are based on capitation, and each Region can decide for itself how to take account of the homeless population in the formula. Some will add to the population base for affected Districts, but do not give a weighting for excess need for health care. There is thus inequity in provision for homeless people.

10 Changing the homeless legislation

In January 1994, the Department of the Environment published a consultation paper the main proposals of which concern the provision of accommodation 'in an emergency' (see Box 7). If these proposals are implemented, they will effectively dismantle the statutory rights currently accorded to people and households who are at present accepted as homeless by local authorities under the provisions of the 1985 (1977) Housing Act. The Government's arguments in support of its proposals are that the current legislation is unfair to people with the same or more housing need, and also that

BOX 7

**Access to local authority and housing association tenancies:
a consultation paper**

Summary of proposals

a   the new duty of an authority will be to assist persons in priority
    need who, through no fault of their own, are without
    accommodation of any sort in an emergency;

b   this duty will start from the time that the authority has established
    the applicant's entitlement;

c   the duty will be to provide accommodation for a limited period;

d   the duty could recur if the household continues to meet all the
    necessary criteria;

e   being asked to leave by friends or relatives will no longer
    automatically confer entitlement to assistance:

f   a person is not entitled to assistance if any sort of suitable
    accommodation – however temporary – is available;

g   a person is not entitled to assistance if he/she could obtain
    alternative accommodation.

The main proposals about the allocation of local authority and
housing association tenancies were:

a   local authorities will allocate all tenancies to persons whose
    names appear on a waiting list that authorities will be obliged to
    keep;

b   authorities' allocation policy must accord with any terms and
    conditions set out in the legislation;

c   local authorities and housing associations should be encouraged
    to maintain joint waiting lists of applicants.

Source: Department of the Environment. *Access to local authority and housing
association tenancies: a consultation paper.* London: DoE, 1994.

the present system is being widely abused.

The Department of the Environment received about 9,000
responses to the consultation paper, the majority of which were
opposed to the changes. The Faculty of Public Health Medicine in
its submission summarised the likely health effects of the proposals
as follows:

If implemented [your proposals] would be likely to increase the risks of ill health among groups of the population who are already at increased risk of disease and premature death.

The proposals are likely to mean that:

Households which already have *excessive* levels of ill health will be given less assurance that they will have their health and housing needs met. Indeed such households are likely to experience increased levels of stress due to the reduced and short-term responsibilities which local authorities will be asked to assume. Households in such a situation may be asked to move after a short-hold assured tenancy has expired and (even assuming the local authority assesses that it still has a responsibility) this pattern of mobility is likely to:

- increase disruption of social networks necessary for relieving social isolation;
- increase stress within the family, increasing risks of domestic violence, child abuse, maternal depression and child behavioural disturbance;
- decrease access to primary care and community health services, decreasing the level of child health surveillance available to children of such households; and
- decrease continuity of care in the community available to such households.
- Increased family disharmony and perhaps violence will occur because access to rehousing via the homelessness route has been blocked. Evidence that households living as licensees of others have increased levels of perceived urgent housing need is contained in the recent DoE sponsored research report.[27]

Regarding the allocation of local authority and housing association tenancies, the Faculty stated:

- The current arrangements for including medical need in the assessment of housing need are ineffective and inadequate. In particular there is evidence for wide-ranging variation in the accessibility of the Medical Priority for Rehousing (MPR) arrangements, and even for those who do gain access to this system there is evidence of inconsistent assessment and outcomes in terms of waiting times and adequacy of rehousing.[25]
- We suggest that the MPR system is currently unable to ensure that health and mobility needs are taken into account in the allocation of housing. This is due to the varying levels of training of medical (and other) assessors but is principally due to the diminished social rented stock which is now available. This stock has become 'residual', that is, it now increasingly contains individuals and households who are disadvantaged in social and economic terms

and the physical nature of the stock (increased proportion of flats) and its location (increased proportion on 'problem estates') are increasing to the level of polarisation in housing—increasingly the situation appears to be that adequate housing is accessible only to those who can afford it.

- Given these circumstances, the proposed guidance on allocations policy should recognise the need to ensure that adequate training and resources be available to local authorities so that they may ensure that individual assessments for community care include assessment of the appropriateness of the individual's housing, and its location, in relation to health and well-being and access to health services and social networks.

POSTSCRIPT

On Monday 18 July 1994 the then Minister of Housing, Sir George Young, announced that the Government proposed to bring before Parliament a Bill that would change the statutory responsibilities of local authorities in respect of their duty to find permanent housing for people who are in priority need and homeless. The proposed arrangements (see Box 7) were to be changed in two respects after the consultation exercise; first, the initial time period during which local authorities would assist those officially accepted as homeless was to be one year, subject to review, and, second, the preferred form of temporary accommodation would be private sector leasing. As this report has made clear, these proposals are considered to be ill-judged and, if implemented, are likely to increase the health risks of homeless people placed in temporary accommodation. It is unfortunate that it may be necessary for the working party to reconvene at a future date to review the new patterns of ill health borne by the 'new' homeless.

References to Chapter 6 appear on page 135.

7 Conclusions

The evidence assembled in this report confirms the relationships between homelessness and ill health. The housing situation is unlikely to improve dramatically in the near future. Although we would support moves to reduce the number of homeless people, at present we are obliged to consider secondary measures which aim to improve access to health care and to establish better monitoring of the effects of homelessness on health. We further recommend an appropriate research programme in this area be developed and funded.

The recommendations made by the many organisations campaigning on behalf of homeless people echo many of those already expressed in other reports into primary health care. In 1981 the Acheson report into primary health care in inner London recognised the need for primary health care team-work to tackle inner city deprivation and recommended that '. . . health authorities and local authorities . . . adopt common areas for which groups of primary care workers are responsible and cooperate in the joint provision of premises . . .' (Para 53).[1] Similarly, more recent studies have highlighted the need for greater flexibility in GP contracts and closer integration of health and social services.[2]

Community care legislation has largely failed to recognise the special needs of homeless people. The few examples of good practice in the delivery of care in the community again emphasise the importance of improved communication and better joint planning and working practices between health, housing, social services and voluntary agencies. The examples set by special schemes such as the HHELP team in east London (Appendix A) are paving the way towards fully integrated services, and the few innovative community care schemes developing appear to have succeeded in spite of, rather than because of, current structures.

There is growing support for the argument that the health problems associated with homelessness are primarily an indicator of the failure of housing policies.[3,4] To date, efforts have been focused on improving access to health and social care, but such special schemes can only have a limited effect on the long-term health profile of homeless people if the root cause of their ill health, homelessness, persists. Sustained improvements in the health status of homeless people can ultimately be achieved only by focusing on both health care provision and improved access to housing.

This health role of housing is now being recognised by some local authorities in their community care and housing policies, but this runs contrary to the central thrust of Government housing policy which has been to encourage the erosion of the subsidised rented sector in favour of wider home-ownership. If homelessness is to be tackled effectively, there must be a restatement of the need for an affordable, acceptable and secure rented sector. The resource implications of increased provision of sheltered, independent and residential accommodation for homeless people are likely to be very considerable, but these costs should be weighed against the extra costs currently being borne by the health sector owing to the higher morbidity, high utilisation and greater readmission rates of homeless people, and, not least, against the unremitting health costs to homeless people themselves.

RECOMMENDATION 7

The Department of Health should introduce systematic monitoring of the health of homeless people and their access to services. This should include:
- principal and secondary health problems
- age and sex
- ethnic mix
- HIV infection, subject to informed consent and pre-screening counselling
- tuberculosis
- GP registration
- hospital admissions
- type of homelessness
- accommodation on discharge.

RECOMMENDATION 8

The NHS Research and Development Directorate should take a lead in commissioning further research on the causes and consequences of all types of homelessness, building on earlier studies.

RECOMMENDATION 9

The Government, through the proposed Regional Offices of the NHS Executive, should take steps to ensure that homeless people are not disadvantaged because of the financial implications of their care for GP fundholders. Although capitation mechanisms should take this into account, in the shorter term, arrangements should be considered that could:

i organise the funding of special practices for homeless people in such a way that these practices would be allowed to administer their own budgets and hence compete with GP fundholders;

ii restructure deprivation payments to GPs, by including a *per capita* payment which incorporates an amount based on the number of homeless people registered at the practice;

iii co-ordinate a nationwide service for handling the medical records of homeless people, thus ensuring that information is transferred smoothly between practices;

iv set national health targets relevant to the health needs of homeless people;

v co-ordinate a national strategy to provide better health care to homeless people.

Such a strategy would permit homeless people to choose where they wish to receive care, either from a non-fundholding practice, a fundholding practice or a special practice.

References to Chapter 7 appear on page 136.

Primary care services for Group II homeless people

The Department of Health has introduced a programme in which 30 primary care projects are now centrally funded. Some of these projects are designed to serve Group I homeless people and others Group II; yet others are aimed at travellers. Some examples of these projects are included in this appendix along with other local initiatives.

Great Chapel Street Medical Centre, London W1, and Wytham Hall Sick Bay, London W9

Established in 1978, the Great Chapel Street walk-in clinic was a pioneer in the provision of special medical services for homeless people. The centre is a branch surgery which receives supplementary financing from a number of sources, and has developed close links with a number of statutory and voluntary organisations.

Staff: The core team consists of three GPs, a practice nurse, a patient care coordinator and an administrator. Surgeries are held by consultant psychiatrists, a chiropodist, a dentist and an optician.

Service delivery: There are daily general practitioner and nurse sessions, with regular supporting specialist sessions. Patients may be referred to drug and alcohol detoxification units and accommodation can be arranged for them in resettlement units.

Uptake of services: In the year 1991–92, 1,425 new patients registered with the service and there were 8,436 consultations.[1]

Special features: Great Chapel Street is part of a network of organisations providing services for homeless people in central London. A visiting psychiatrist attends the local magistrate's court weekly to assess the mental state of defendants suspected of suffering from mental illness, prior to their hearing. They may be referred to Great Chapel Street for psychiatric supervision. Those awaiting trial may be referred to the 'bail bed' at Wytham Hall for supervision.

Wytham Hall

The 14-bed sick bay at Wytham Hall was established in 1983 to provide convalescent care, rehabilitation and rehousing for sick homeless people.

Staff: A number of doctors based in hospitals and at the Great Chapel Street Centre provide 24-hour medical cover on a voluntary basis. The social care, rehabilitation and housing needs of patients are managed by two full-time administrators.

Service delivery: The activities of Wytham Hall are illustrated by the diagram opposite (reproduced from the annual report for 1991–1992).[2]

Primary Care for Homeless People (PCHP)

In 1986 the Department of Health funded pilot schemes in two FHSAs (Camden and Islington, and City and East London) to provide medical care and to assist with access to mainstream services for Group II homeless people. Following an evaluation of these projects by the Policy Studies Institute (Williams and Allen 1990), these projects were modified and the initiative was extended to a further 10 FHSAs.

East London Homeless Primary Care Team (HHELP)

This project aims to provide medical services to Group II homeless people and facilitate their integration into mainstream services.

Staff: The original team was led by a salaried GP. This was not satisfactory because he did not have the links with mainstream providers necessary to facilitate integration. The salaried GP was therefore replaced by eight local GPs working with the primary health care team on a sessional basis.

The project has developed joint funding arrangements with a number of bodies to employ social workers, clinical nurse specialists, a clinical psychologist and others. HHELP collaborates with the Homeless Mentally Ill (HMI) initiative which was announced in 1990 to serve severely mentally ill people sleeping rough in central London, and provides a 20-bed residential unit. When this initiative is complete, it will provide 149 beds across London.

NETWORK OF SERVICES CENTRED AROUND WYTHAM HALL

WYTHAM HALL

COURT DIVERSION SCHEME
for mentally ill offenders

Consultant psychiatrist attends magistrate's court weekly to assess the mental state of offenders suspected of suffering with a mental illness, before their initial hearing. May be referred to the Wytham Hall bail bed or continue psychiatric supervision at Great Chapel Street if they are released.

NOTTING HILL GATE SURGERY

Patients referred from Wytham Hall for regular appointments for eg psychotherapy, dietary advice, and to register after discharge, if appropriate.

GREAT CHAPEL STREET MEDICAL CENTRE

Patients are referred, where necessary, to Wytham Hall, local hospitals or specialist services eg housing, alcohol advice and detoxification etc. Patients continue to see a doctor here after discharge from Wytham Hall.

HOUSING AND FOLLOW-UP

All patients are discharged to housing and have follow-up support:
- Bed & Breakfast via homeless persons unit
- Hostels
- Supportive housing
- Residential care homes
- Bedsits and flats through Westminster Council and Central Government Rough Sleepers Initiative
- Plans underway to set up a shared house, where patients can live as a community.

COLD WEATHER SHELTERS

Weekly clinics held at selected Cold Weather Shelters during the months they are open. Most problems are dealt with immediately but some may warrant referral to other services, including Wytham Hall and Great Chapel Street.

ST MARTIN-IN-THE-FIELDS

Day centre and social care unit. Twice weekly surgeries held here since 1983. Patients may be referred to Wytham Hall or Great Chapel Street for treatment.

LOCAL HOSPITALS

Increasing numbers of patients are referred to Wytham Hall on discharge for convalescent care and medical supervision. Patients are referred from Wytham Hall for specialist investigation and/or treatment.

REFERRALS MADE TO SERVICES

Dentist, optician, alcohol advice and counselling, day centres, housing etc. Day care: wood workshops, printing, adult education classes, day hospital.

Source of Referrals to Wytham Hall 1991–1992

Mobile Surgery 5
Local Hospitals 22
St Martins 18
Other agencies 20
GCS 94

Source: Wytham Hall Annual Report 1991–1992

Methods of working: Both the primary health care and HMI teams contact patients through outreach work on the streets and through sessions in a number of local day centres and hostels for homeless people. The HMI team also holds sessions in Holloway prison and with the east London women's group Access.

Uptake of services: In 1991/92 the HHELP team had almost 7,000 individual consultations. The majority of people seen by the team are male (70%) but the team attempts to contact women through weekly women's groups and sessions at local women's hostels.[3]

Special features: The service aims particularly to provide advocacy services to assist patients with rehousing.

Primary Health Care Project for Homeless People in Bristol

This project was established in February 1992 to provide comprehensive general medical services for Group II homeless people.

Staff: The primary health care team consists of two GPs from a local health centre, a salaried GP, a full-time nurse, a part-time nurse specialising in mental health and a clerical officer/receptionist.

Service delivery: The team holds five sessions a week in two different centres. Nurses conduct outreach work with people living on the streets and provide information about the primary health care project. The team works closely with local voluntary and statutory organisations.

Uptake of services: 806 consultations were made by 321 individuals between April and September 1992. Forty-seven per cent of users claimed to be registered with a GP, and a further 23 clients were helped to register. Less than 10% of the users were women.[4]

Special features: The team has attempted to introduce portable patient-held treatment records to facilitate continuity of care between providers. Despite the advantages of such cards, uptake has so far been poor (8%).

Nottingham Homelessness Projects

A number of services are available for homeless people in Nottingham but until recently they have been largely uncoordinated. A multi-agency working party has been set up to develop a strategy for health care for homeless people in the district. The services currently provided in the city include:

1. Community Health Team for the Homeless

Aim: To provide homeless people with access to primary nursing care, counselling and support and mainstream services.

Staff: The team consists of two liaison nurses for single homeless people, and a liaison nurse, midwife and health visitor for homeless families, pregnant women and young people.

Service delivery: The community liaison nurse for single homeless people provides primary nursing care through walk-in clinics, and screening and monitoring for individuals at risk. Alcohol and drug abuse, mental health and health services are provided. The nurse liaises with other statutory, voluntary and private agencies. The team also aims to act as a resource for research and development by collecting information and data relating to the specific needs of homeless people.

2. Mental Health Support Team Nottingham

Aim: To provide counselling and support to single homeless people with mental health or substance abuse problems, and to improve their access to mental health services.

Staff: Two social workers and two workers for the homeless, together with other workers with expertise in mental health.

Service delivery: The team liaises with local agencies and provides support and training to hostel workers and other staff in contact with mentally ill people.

Uptake of the service: During the year March 1992 to March 1993 the team dealt with 207 new cases of which about half were short-term referrals (requiring anything from an assessment visit to more intensive support for a few weeks) and half long-term referrals. The team also continued to support 56 ongoing cases from previous years. Ninety per cent of these referrals came from hostels and night shelters for homeless people. (Nottingham Hostels Liaison Group Update, April 1993.)

3. General practitioners

Two practices agree to see homeless people at their surgeries without an appointment and also provide sessions at different hostels in the district.

Leeds Health Care Team for the Homeless and Rootless

Aim: This team, established in 1989 aims to integrate the homeless and hostel population (Group II) into primary health care services where appropriate, and to provide ongoing medical care when this is not possible.

Staff: The team comprises a salaried GP, a practice nurse, a community psychiatric nurse, a liaison worker and a secretary.

Service delivery: The team holds 14 clinic sessions per week in various hostels and day centres for homeless people across the city. Weekly clinics are also held at the city detoxification unit and at the resettlement unit. The team will also see people in other locations (eg on the street) when necessary. The salaried GP has a prescribing budget and can make referrals in the usual way but cannot register patients or provide 24-hour cover.

Uptake of the service: During the year July 1991–July 1992 the team dealt with 3,418 consultations.[5]

Special features: A multi-agency single access point in Leeds city centre is planned.

Luther Street Centre, Oxford

The Luther Street Centre, based in Oxford city centre, was established in 1985 as a health and advice centre. Originally operating as a branch surgery, it became a directly funded unit in July 1992. It aims to provide medical advice and support services for homeless people who are not registered with a local GP and find it difficult to gain access to traditional services and to help them achieve a more stable lifestyle. The groups served include both Group I and Group II homeless categories as well as squatters and New Age travellers.

Staff: The project team comprises two medical directors (job sharing), a project director/trust administrator, a nurse/outreach worker, a part-time practice nurse, a twilight hours practice nurse and a reception team. Regular clinics are provided by alcohol and drug workers, a chiropodist, an acupuncturist, counsellors and a psychiatric registrar.

Service delivery: The GPs hold open access surgeries each weekday morning. Domiciliary sessions are given at a local hostel, occasional sessions are held at travellers' sites within the county and other outreach services are offered. In addition to general medical services, the team also provides advice, advocacy and broker services to patients. Health promotion activities include HIV/AIDS testing, counselling, needle exchange and the provision of free condoms.

Uptake of the service: In the year to 31 March 1993 a total of 10,100 consultations were made with 1,076 people. Of these, 62% were suffering from alcohol problems, 27% from drug abuse and 24% from chronic mental illness. Women accounted for less than 11% of users.[6]

Special features: Efforts are currently being made to carry out a national survey of health care needs and provision for homeless people.

Hanover Project Sheffield

This three-year project funded by the Department of Health and Trent RHA was established to provide extra resources to meet the health care needs of homeless people in Sheffield. It aims to improve the standard of care offered to homeless people by integrating their care into the established primary care system.

Staff: The project involves a GP practice of six partners (3 full-time and 3 part-time) together with three part-time practice nurses, two full-time health visitors (devoting 25% of their time exclusively to homeless people), a community psychiatric nurse (50% homeless), a part-time alcohol counsellor (6 hours per week) and a general counsellor (7 hours per week). A social worker, chiropodist and consultant psychiatrist are also involved.

Service delivery: The project operates as a regular GP partnership serving all those residing within the practice area (ie Groups I and II as well as the general population). Homeless people presenting at the centre are offered permanent or temporary registration, whichever is most suited to their situation. The project health visitors and the community psychiatric nurse visit a range of home-less 'residences' including hotels housing homeless families. They provide nursing care, counselling and advice and also encourage appropriate use of the GP surgery. Health checks are offered to all new patients registering with the practice. Good uptake of this service has led to the detection of many asymptomatic conditions such as high blood pressure and diabetes.

Special features: The project has been successful in developing an integrated service, thanks to the commitment to accept homeless people and to the practical allocation of special funds for the necessary additional staff.[7]

References to the Appendices appear on page 137.

APPENDIX B
Services for Group I homeless families

Bayswater Centre

During the 1980s Bayswater became a common destination for homeless families from other London boroughs. The Bayswater Centre houses four types of service for homeless families:

- the Bayswater Hotel Homelessness Project provides advocacy services for families experiencing difficulties in gaining access to local services
- the Bayswater Family Centre offers play space for children and a meeting place for parents
- the Bayswater Care Team consists of specialist health visitors and social workers
- the Bayswater Families Doctors Practice (BFDP).[8]

Staff: The BFDP consists of 16 local GPs working on a rota, a full-time nurse, a practice manager and a receptionist.

Service delivery: The BFDP operates as a branch surgery of a local practice. Sixteen local GPs work on a rota offering two-hour surgeries every afternoon. The practice nurse offers appointments outside GP surgery hours, smear tests, immunisations, vaccinations, registration checks and health promotion clinics. Given the constant change of personnel on the GP rota, the practice nurse plays an important role in ensuring continuity of care.

Uptake of the service: There were 4,047 consultations at the BFDP between July 1991 and June 1992.

Nottingham Community Health Team for Homeless Families, Women and Young People

Aim: This team aims to provide homeless people with access to primary nursing care, counselling and support, and referral to mainstream services.

119

Staff: The team consists of a nurse, a midwife and a health visitor.

Service delivery: The team offers primary health care, midwifery, pregnancy testing, health visiting and health promotion clinics.

Marylebone Health Centre

Aim: This mainstream general practice was established in 1987 and emphasises 'a multidisciplinary approach to whole person care'.

Staff: The team includes three GPs and a full-time practice nurse, with support from a health visitor, a community psychiatric nurse, a community midwife and a district nurse.

Service delivery: The GP practice registers homeless families on a permanent basis, provides primary care and also makes referrals to a number of complementary medical practitioners.

Uptake of the service: In the year December 1991 to December 1992 the outreach worker saw a total of 82 families, representing 225 family members; 120 people were within families living in bed and breakfast hotels. A high proportion (75%) of these families were immigrants and refugees from a wide range of countries including Bangladesh, Nigeria, Somalia, Zaïre and the former Yugoslavia. The majority of the problems for which clients were referred related to housing (65%) and social security benefits (31%). Health problems (26%) typically were a result of unsatisfactory accommodation and high levels of stress.[9]

Tower Hamlets Specialist Health Visitor for Homeless Families

This project has set up a system whereby health visitors are notified when a homeless family moves on to their 'patch'. The specialist health visitor offers training sessions for health visitors and other NHS staff to break down negative stereotypes, explain the causes of homelessness and the problems faced by homeless people, and to provide information about resources available to homeless people.

References to the Appendices appear on page 137.

Examples of good practice in discharge arrangements

London Borough of Southwark

The London Borough of Southwark has developed a scheme whereby people due for discharge from hospital are given the same priority as those in other forms of temporary accommodation. The social worker obtains evidence of vulnerability direct from hospital doctors, thus increasing the possibility that suitable accommodation will be found before the person is discharged.

Albert Hotel Scheme, St Mary's Hospital, London

The Albert Hotel Scheme, run by St Mary's Hospital, London, aims to provide residential home/social services type accommodation for low-dependency patients who are fit for discharge from hospital but, for various reasons (which may or may not include homeless-ness), cannot return home. The 'hotel's' operational policy[10] states that:

> 'Acute ward staff must demonstrate that they have made every effort to facilitate discharge and identify ongoing support or facilities. It is only when the ongoing support is not available that the hospital hotel will admit.'

Admission to the hotel allows time to arrange suitable care and accommodation and enables high-care beds in the hospital to be used more efficiently.

References to the Appendices appear on page 137.

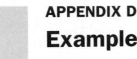

APPENDIX D

Examples of good practice in joint planning and services

London Borough of Haringey

A joint project of the departments of housing and social services in the London Borough of Haringey provides accommodation in a short-term hostel with 24 bedsits for homeless people who are vulnerable due to mental ill health. It is staffed by officers from both departments who make a full assessment of accommodation and support services needs. Referrals to the hostel are made through the homeless persons unit. (CHAR 1993.)

London Borough of Greenwich

The housing department of the London Borough of Greenwich runs two projects on similar lines which cater for all vulnerable people, not just those suffering from mental ill health. One of the projects provides temporary independent bedsit accommodation for women only and has a small amount of space for women with children.

Other London Authorities

A number of London authorities (including Waltham Forest, Kingston and Enfield) have established vulnerability panels made up of representatives from housing and social services and, in some cases, the health authority and voluntary sector. Although these panels have varying remits, they usually function as a decision making body to assess applications made by homeless people with mental illness, learning difficulties or other special problems. The panels consider medical and social reports and decide whether the person can be considered vulnerable under the terms of the Housing Act. The advantage of this approach is that it promotes closer working relationships between housing and social services departments. Since the panel assesses both housing and support needs in the beginning, applicants are also more likely to be placed in appropriate housing.

West End Central Police Station

Group II homeless people, especially street dwellers, frequently come into contact with the police who may, in the discharge of their duties, identify individuals with acute or chronic health problems or who are in urgent need of shelter. At West End Central Police Station, some officers have been given specific responsibility for matters relating to homeless people in their area and have established good working relationships with the local statutory authorities (health and local authority) and voluntary agencies.

References to the Appendices appear on page 137.

References

Chapter 1: **Definitions, statistics and context of homelessness**

1. *Inequalities in health: the Black report and the health divide.* Harmondsworth: Penguin Books, 1988.
2. Department of Health. *The Health of the Nation: a strategy for health in England.* London: HMSO, 1992 (Cmnd 1986).
3. Health Promotion Authority for Wales. *Health for all in Wales: strategies for action* (Parts A, B and C). Cardiff: HPAW, 1990.
4. Scottish Office. *Scotland's health: a challenge to us all.* Edinburgh: HMSO, 1992.
5. DHSS Northern Ireland. *A regional strategy for Northern Ireland health and personal social services, 1992–1997.* Belfast: DHSS-NI, 1992.
6. World Health Organisation. *'Health for all': the health policy for Europe.* Copenhagen: WHO, 1993.
7. Connelly J, Kelleher C, Morton S, St James D, Roderick P. *Housing or homelessness: a public health perspective,* 2nd edn. London: Faculty of Public Health Medicine, 1992.
8. Bramley G, Doogan K, Leather P, Murie A, Watson E, eds. *Homelessness and the London housing market.* Bristol: School for Advanced Urban Studies, 1988.
9. Pahl J, Vaile M. *Health and health care among travellers.* Maidstone Health Authority and the Health Services Research Unit, University of Kent, Canterbury, 1986.
10. Hussey R. Travellers and preventive health care: what are health authorities doing? *British Medical Journal* 1988; **296**: 1098.
11. Feder G. Traveller gypsies and primary care. *Journal of the Royal College of General Practitioners* 1989; **39**: 425–9.
12. Feder G, Hussey R. Traveller mothers and babies. *British Medical Journal* 1990; **300**: 1536–7.
13. Audit Commission. *Housing the homeless: the local authority role.* London: HMSO, 1989.
14. Department of the Environment, Welsh Office, Scottish Development Office. *Households accepted as homeless* (Quarterly).
15. Anderson I, Kemp P, Quilgars D. *Single homeless people.* London: HMSO, 1993.
16. Fisher K, Collins J, eds. *Homelessness, health care and welfare provision.* London: Routledge, 1993.
17. Austerberry H, Watson S. *Women on the margins.* London: City University Housing Research Group, 1983.
18. Morris J, Winn M. *Housing and social inequality.* London: Hilary Shipman, 1990.
19. Office of Population Censuses and Surveys. *Communal establishments:*

Census 1991. London: HMSO, 1993.

20. Moore J, Canter D, Stockley D, Drake M. *Faces of homelessness.* Housing Research Unit, Department of Psychology, University of Surrey, 1991.
21. Shelter's 25th anniversary report. *Building for the future.* London: Shelter, 1991.
22. Randall G. Out for the count. *Roof* 1993; Oct/Nov.
23. Fisher N, Turner SW, Pugh R, Taylor C. Estimating numbers of homeless and homeless mentally ill people in north east Westminster by using capture-recapture analysis. *British Medical Journal* 1994; **308**: 27–30.
24. Garside PL, Grimshaw RW, Ward FJ. *No place like home: the hostels experience.* London: HMSO, 1990.
25. Official record of Parliament. *Hansard* 27 February 1991, cols 961–3.
26. Strathdee R. *Housing our children: the Children Act 1989.* London: Centrepoint Soho, 1993.
27. Drake J, Conway J, Holman C, Buckley K. *Homes for our children: a report from the National Housing Forum.* London: NHF, 1992.
28. Niner P. *Housing needs in the 1990s: an interim assessment.* National Housing Forum. London: National Federation of Housing Associations, 1989.
29. Department of the Environment. *National dwelling and housing survey.* London: HMSO, 1979.
30. Green H, Holroyd S. *Shared accommodation in England, 1990.* OPCS. London: HMSO, 1992.
31. Clapham D, Kemp P, Smith SJ, eds. *Housing and social policy.* London: Macmillan, 1990.
32. LeGrand S, Robinson R, eds. *Privatisation and the welfare state.* London: Allen and Unwin, 1984.
33. Berthoud R, ed. *Challenges to social policy.* Aldershot: Gower, 1985.
34. Hills J. *The future of welfare: a guide to the debate.* York: Joseph Rowntree Foundation, 1993.
35. Greve J. *Homelessness in Britain.* York: Joseph Rowntree Foundation, 1991.
36. Lambert C, Jeffers S, Burton P, Bramley G. *Homelessness in rural areas.* Rural Development Commission, 1992.
37. Whitehead C, Kleinmann M. *A review of housing needs assessment.* London: Housing Corporation, 1992.
38. Maclennan D, Williams R, eds. *Affordable housing in Europe.* York: Joseph Rowntree Foundation, 1990.
39. Maclennan D, Williams R, eds. *Housing subsidies and the market: an international perspective.* York: Joseph Rowntree Foundation, 1990.
40. National Federation of Housing Associations. *Inquiry into British housing,* chaired by the Duke of Edinburgh. Second report, 1991.
41. Murie A. *Housing inequality and deprivation.* London: Heinemann, 1983.
42. Bramley G. *Bridging the affordability gap in the 1990s: an update of research on housing access and affordability.* Birmingham: BEC Publications, 1991.
43. Foster S. *Missing the target.* London: Shelter, 1992.

44. *Filling England's empty homes.* Housing research findings, No. 111. York: Joseph Rowntree Foundation, 1994.
45. Bramley G. *Meeting housing needs.* London: Association of District Councils, 1989.
46. Bramley G. The demand for social housing in England in the 1980s. *Housing Studies* 1989; **4**(1): 18–35.
47. Department of the Environment. *Access to local authority and housing association tenancies: a consultation paper.* London: DoE, 1994.
48. Royal Society of Health Conference, Manchester, March 1994. Conference papers. *Health aspects of housing estates.*

Chapter 2: Health and housing opportunities

1. Smith SJ. Health status and the housing system. *Social Science and Medicine* 1990; **31**(7): 753–62.
2. Clapham D, Kemp P, Smith SJ, eds. *Housing and social policy.* London: Macmillan, 1990.
3. Connelly J, Kelleher C, Morton S, St James D, Roderick P. *Housing or homelessness: a public health perspective.* London: Faculty of Public Health Medicine, 1992.
4. Morris J, Winn M. *Housing and social inequality.* London: Hilary Shipman, 1991.
5. Shelter's 25th anniversary report. *Building for the future.* London: Shelter, 1991.
6. Department of the Environment. *Homelessness statistics.* Annually.
7. *Debt and credit survey.* London: Policy Studies Institute, 1992.
8. *Housing trailers to 1981 and 1984 labour force survey.* London: HMSO, 1988.
9. Association of District Councils. *Survey on council house rents, housing subsidy and capital expenditure.* London: Association of District Councils, 1990.
10. Audit Commission. *Survey of local authority housing rent arrears.* London: HMSO, 1989.
11. Evans A, Duncan S. *Responding to homelessness: local authority policy and practice.* London: HMSO, 1989.
12. *Inequalities in health: the Black report and the health divide.* Harmondsworth: Penguin Books, 1988.
13. Townsend P, Phillmore P, Beattie A. *Health and deprivation.* London: Routledge, 1989.
14. Delamothe T. Social inequalities in health. *British Medical Journal* 1991; **303**: 1046–50.
15. Smith R. *Unemployment and health.* Oxford: Oxford University Press, 1988.
16. Bartley M. Health and labour force participation. *Journal of Social Policy* 1991; **20**: 3–10.
17. Fox AJ, Goldblatt PO. *Longitudinal study: socio-demographic mortality differentials.* OPCS series LS No. 1. London: HMSO, 1982.
18. Fagin L, Little M. *The forsaken families: the effects of unemployment on*

family life. Harmondsworth: Penguin Books, 1984.

19. Warr P. Job-loss, unemployment and psychological well-being. In: Allen VL, van de Vliert E, eds. *Role transitions: explorations and explanations.* New York, London: Plenum Press, 1984.

20. Watchman PO, Robson P. *Homelessness and the law in Britain.* Glasgow: Planning Exchange, 1989.

21. Shanks N, Smith SJ. British public policy and the health of homeless people. *Policy and Politics* 1992; **20**(1): 35–46.

22. Smith SJ, Knill-Jones R, McGuckin A, eds. *Housing for health.* London: Longman, 1991.

23. Sunkin M. An appealing idea. *Housing* 1988; March: 14.

24. Prescott-Clarke P, Clemens S, Park A. *Routes into local authority housing: a study of local authority waiting lists and new tenancies.* Department of the Environment. London: HMSO, 1994.

25. Smith SJ, McGuckin A, Hill S, Alexander A. *Housing provision for people with health problems and mobility difficulties.* Five reports available from Smith SJ, Department of Geography, University of Edinburgh. Summary available as *Housing research findings* No. 86. York: Joseph Rowntree Foundation, 1993.

26. Audit Commission. *Developing local authority housing strategies.* London: HMSO, 1992.

27. Audit Commission. *Housing the homeless: the local authority role.* London: HMSO, 1989.

28. Roderick P, Victor CR, Connelly J. Is housing a public health issue? A survey of directors of public health. *British Medical Journal* 1991; **302**: 157–60.

Chapter 3: Health problems of homeless families

1. Department of the Environment. *Homelessness statistics.* Reported annually.

2. Audit Commission Report. *Housing the homeless: the local authority role.* London: HMSO, 1989.

3. Connelly J, Kelleher C, Morton S, St James D, Roderick P. *Housing or homelessness: a public health perspective.* London: Faculty of Public Health Medicine, 1992.

4. Victor CR. Health status of the temporarily homeless population and residents of North West Thames Region. *British Medical Journal* 1992; **305**: 387–91.

5. Mant D. Understanding the problems of health and housing research. In: Burridge R, Ormandy D, eds. *Unhealthy housing: research, remedies and reform.* London: E&FN Spon, 1993.

6. Drennan V, Stearn J. Health visitors and homeless families. *Health Visitor* 1986; **59**(11): 340–2.

7. Stearn J. An expensive way of making children ill. *Roof* 1986; Sept/Oct: 11–4.

8. Lovell B. Health visiting homeless families. *Health Visitor* 1986; **59**(11): 334–7.

9. Parsons L. Homeless families in Hackney. *Public Health* 1991; **105**: 287–96.
10. Conway J, Kemp P. *Bed and breakfast.* London: SHAC, 1985.
11. Conway J, ed. *Prescription for poor health: the crisis for homeless families.* London: London Food Commission, Maternity Alliance, SHAC, Shelter, 1988.
12. Murie A, Jaffers S. *The experience of bed and breakfast living.* Bristol: School for Advanced Urban Studies, 1990.
13. Heaton PA, Charlton TL. Burns affecting children from homeless families. *Journal of Maternal and Child Health* 1993; **18**: 16–21.
14. Health Visitors Association and General Medical Services Committee of BMA. *Homeless families and their health.* London: HVA/BMA, 1989.
15. HM Inspectorate of Schools. *A survey of the education of children living in temporary accommodation.* Department of Education and Science. London: HMSO, 1990.
16. Vickers M. *Health and living conditions of homeless families in Oxford city: literature review and analysis of collected data.* Oxford District Health Authority Community Unit/Oxford City Council Environmental Health Department. Unpublished report, 1991.
17. Victor CR, Connelly J, Roderick P, Cohen C. Use of hospital services by homeless families in an inner London health district. *British Medical Journal* 1989; **299**: 725–7.
18. Lissauer T, Richman S, Tempia M, Jenkins S, Taylor B. Influence of homelessness on acute admissions to hospital. *Archives of Disease in Childhood* 1993; **69**: 423–9.
19. Richman S, Roderick P, Victor CR, Lissauer T. Use of acute hospital services by homeless children. *Public Health* 1991; **105**: 297–302.
20. Patterson CM, Roderick P. Obstetric outcome in homeless women. *British Medical Journal* 1990; **301**: 263–6.
21. Barker DJP, ed. *Infant origins of adult disease.* London: British Medical Journal Books, 1992.
22. Thomas A, Niner P. *Living in temporary accommodation: survey of homeless people.* Department of the Environment. London: HMSO, 1989: 121, 124.

Chapter 4: **The health of single homeless people**

1. Wright JD, Weber E. *Homelessness and health.* Washington: McGraw-Hill, 1987.
2. Shanks NJ. Mortality among inmates of a common lodging house. *Journal of the Royal College of General Practitioners* 1984; **34**: 38–40.
3. Keyes S, Kennedy M. *Sick to death of homelessness.* London: Crisis, 1992.
4. Deaths among homeless persons—Georgia. *Morbidity and Mortality Weekly Report* 1987; **36**: 297–9.
5. Deaths among homeless persons—San Francisco, 1985–1990. *Morbidity and Mortality Weekly Report* 1991; **42**: 605.
6. Hibbs JR, Benner L, Klugman L, Spencer R, Macchia I, Mellinger AK, Fife D. Mortality in a cohort of homeless adults in Philadelphia. *New*

England Journal of Medicine 1994; **331**: 304–9.

7. Alstrom CH, Lindelious R, Salum I. Mortality among homeless men. *British Journal of Addiction* 1975; **70**: 245–52.

8. George SL, Shanks NJ, Westlake L. Census of single homeless people in Sheffield. *British Medical Journal* 1991; **302**: 1387–9.

9. Bines W. *The health of single homeless people.* York University Centre for Housing Policy, 1994.

10. Whynes DK, Giggs JA. The health of the Nottingham homeless. *Public Health* 1992; **106**: 307–14.

11. Shanks NJ. Medical morbidity of the homeless. *Journal of Epidemiology and Community Health* 1988; **42**: 183–6.

12. Balazs J. Health care for the single homeless. In: Fisher K, ed. *Homelessness, health care and welfare provision.* London: Routledge, 1993.

13. Toon PD, Thomas K, Doherty M. Audit of work at a medical centre for the homeless over one year. *Journal of the Royal College of General Practitioners* 1987; **37**: 120–2.

14. Gaskell PG. MD thesis, Glasgow University, 1969.

15. Braddick MR, Thompson MM. Destitution at the Festive Season. *Lancet* 1989; **i**: 330.

16. Powell P. A 'house-doctor' scheme for primary health care for single homeless in Edinburgh. *Journal of the Royal College of General Practitioners* 1987; **37**: 444–7.

17. Shanks NJ. Medical provision for the homeless in Manchester. *Journal of the Royal College of General Practitioners* 1983; **33**: 40–3.

18. Ramsden SS, Nyiri P, Bridgewater J, El-Kabir DJ. A mobile surgery for single homeless people in London. *British Medical Journal* 1989; **298**: 372–4.

19. Scott R, Gaskell PG, Morrell DC. Patients who reside in common lodging houses. *British Medical Journal* 1966; **ii**: 1561–4.

20. Lodge-Patch IC. Homeless men in London. 1. Demographic findings in a lodging house sample. *British Journal of Psychiatry* 1971; **118**: 313–7.

21. Morrell DC. The Edinburgh common lodging house: a challenge in medical care. *Scottish Medical Journal* 1967; **12**: 171–7.

22. Featherstone P, Ashmore C. Health surveillance project among single homeless men in Bristol. *Journal of the Royal College of General Practitioners* 1988; **38**: 353–5.

23. Breakey W, Fischer P, Kramer M, Neustadt G, Romanoski A, Ross A, Royall R, Stine O. Health and mental health problems of homeless men and women in Baltimore. *Journal of the American Medical Association* 1989; **262**: 1352–7.

24. Connelly J, Kelleher C, Morton S, St James D, Roderick P. *Housing or homelessness: a public health perspective,* 2nd edn. London: Faculty of Public Health Medicine, 1992.

25. Dunne FJ. Alcohol abuse on skid row: in sight and out of mind. *Alcohol and Alcoholism* 1990; **25**: 13–5.

26. Rotheram-Borus MJ. Homeless youths and HIV infection. *American Psychologist* 1991; **46**: 1188–97.

27. Marshall EJ, Reed JL. Psychiatric morbidity in homeless women. *British Journal of Psychiatry* 1991; **160**: 761–9.

28. Bramley G, Doogan K, Leather P, Murie A, Watson E, eds. *Homelessness and the London housing market.* Bristol: School for Advanced Urban Studies, 1988.

29. Stephens D, Dennie E, Toomer M, Holloway J. The diversity of case management needs for the care of homeless persons. *Public Health Reports* 1991; **106**: 15–9.

30. Mercat A, Nguyen J, Dantzenberg B. An outbreak of pneumococcal pneumonia in two men's shelters. Chest 1991; 99: 147–51.

31. De Maria A. Pneumococcal pneumonia in a men's shelter. *Journal of the American Medical Association* 1980; **244**: 1446.

32. Gelberg L, Linn LS, Usatine RP, Smith MH. Health, homelessness and poverty: a study of clinic users. *Archives of Internal Medicine* 1990; **150**: 2325–30.

33. Collett DN. *Annual practice report, 1992.* Luther Street Centre, Oxford.

34. Watson JM. Tuberculosis in Britain today [editorial]. *British Medical Journal* 1993; **306**: 221–2.

35. Salpeter S. Tuberculosis chemoprophylaxis [see comments]. *Western Journal of Medicine* (San Francisco) 1992; **157**: 421–4.

36. Tuberculosis among pregnant women—New York City, 1985–1992. *Morbidity and Mortality Weekly Report* 1993; **42**: 605–12.

37. Rosenfield EA, Hageman JR, Yogev R. Tuberculosis in infancy in the 1990s. *Pediatric Clinics of North America* 1993; **40**: 1087–103.

38. Raviglione MC, Sudre P, Rieder HL, Spinaci S, Kochi A. Secular trends of tuberculosis in Western Europe. *Bulletin of the World Health Organisation* 1993; **71**: 297–306.

39. Bakshi SS, Alvarez D, Hilfer CL, Sordillo EM, Grover R, Kairam R. Tuberculosis in human immunodeficiency virus-infected children: a family infection. *American Journal of Diseases of Children* 1993; **147**: 320–4.

40. Davies PD. Tuberculosis is increasing in England and Wales [letter]. *British Medical Journal* 1993; **307**: 63.

41. Symonds JM. Incidence of tuberculosis in England and Wales: Europeans may be more at risk [letter]. *British Medical Journal* 1993; **307**: 866.

42. Lerner BH. New York City's tuberculosis control efforts: the historical limitations of the 'war on consumption'. *American Journal of Public Health* 1993; **83**: 758–66.

43. Genewein A, Telenti A, Bernasconi C, Mordaasini C, Weiss S, Maurer AM, Reider HL, Schopfer K, Bodmer T. Molecular approach to identifying route of transmission of tuberculosis in the community [see comments]. *Lancet* 1993; **342**: 817–8.

44. Ramsden SS, Baur S, El-Kabir DJ. TB among the central London single homeless. *Journal of the Royal College of Physicians of London* 1988; **22**: 16–7.

45. Patel KR. Pulmonary tuberculosis in residents of lodging houses, night shelters and common hostels in Glasgow: a five year prospective survey. *British Journal of Diseases of the Chest* 1985; **79**: 60–6.

46. Hellman SL, Gram MC. The resurgence of tuberculosis: risk in health care settings. *AAOHN Journal* 1993; **41**: 66–72.

47. Centers for Disease Control. TB among homeless shelter residents. *Journal of the American Medical Association* 1992; **267**: 483–4.

48. Wosornu D, MacIntyre D, Watt B. An outbreak of isoniazid resistant tuberculosis in Glasgow, 1981–88. *Respiratory Medicine* 1990; **84**: 361–4.

49. Etkind S, Ford J, Nardell E, Boutotte J, Singleton L. Treating 'hard-to-treat' TB patients in Massachusetts. *Seminars in Respiratory Infections* 1991; **6**: 273–82.

50. Citron KM, Girling DJ. Tuberculosis. In: Weatherall DJ, Ledingham JGG, Warrell DA, eds. *Oxford textbook of medicine*, 2nd edn. Oxford: Oxford University Press, 1987: 5.278–5.299.

51. Caplin M, Rehahn M. Alcoholism and tuberculosis. In: Vere DW, ed. *Topics in therapeutics*, 4. London: Royal College of Physicians, 1978: 136–49.

52. Capewell S, France AJ, Anderson M, Leitch AG. The diagnosis and management of tuberculosis in common hostel dwellers. *Tubercle* 1986; **67**: 125–31.

53. Drucker E. Molecular epidemiology meets the fourth world [comment]. *Lancet* 1993; **342**: 817–8.

54. Torres RA, Mani S, Altholz J, Brickner PW. HIV infection among homeless men in a New York shelter. *Archives of Internal Medicine* 1990; **150**: 2030–6.

55. Hayward C. Re-emergence of tuberculosis [letter]. *British Medical Journal* 1993; **306**: 515.

56. Springett VH, Watson JM. Re-emergence of tuberculosis [letter]. *British Medical Journal* 1993; **306**: 932.

57. Citron KM. BCG vaccination against tuberculosis: international perspectives [editorial]. *British Medical Journal* 1993; **306**: 222–3.

58. Davies PD. Control of communicable disease: tuberculosis screening falls foul of reforms [letter]. *British Medical Journal* 1993; **307**: 59.

59. Bayer R, Dubler NN, Landesman S. The dual epidemics of tuberculosis and AIDS: ethical and policy issues in screening and treatment. *American Journal of Public Health* 1993; **83**: 649–54.

60. Wrenn K. Foot problems in homeless persons. *Annals of Internal Medicine* 1990; **113**: 567–9.

61. Scharer KL, Berson A, Brickner PW. Lack of housing and its impact on human health: a service perspective. *Bulletin of the New York Academy of Medicine* 1990; **66**: 515–25.

62. Reed R, Ramsden S, Marshall J, Ball J, O'Brien J, Flynn A, Elton N, El-Kabir D, Joseph P. Psychiatric morbidity and substance abuse among residents of a cold weather shelter. *British Medical Journal* 1992; **304**: 1028–9.

63. Fisher PJ. Estimating the prevalence of alcohol, drug and mental health problems in the contemporary homeless population. *Contemporary Drug Problems* 1989; **16**: 333–9.

64. McCarty D, Argeriou M, Heubner RB, Lubrau B. Alcoholism, drug abuse and the homeless. *American Psychologist* 1991; **46**: 1139–48.

65. Anderson I, Kemp P, Quilgars D. *Single homeless people*. Department of the Environment. London: HMSO, 1993.

Chapter 5: Mental health and homelessness

1. Scott J. Homelessness and mental illness. *British Journal of Psychiatry* 1993; **162**: 314–25.
2. Cohen NL, Putnam JF, Sullivan AM. The mentally ill homeless: isolation and adaptation. *Hospital and Community Psychiatry* 1984; **35**: 922–4.
3. Bines W. *The health of single homeless people*. York University Centre for Housing Policy, 1994.
4. Tidmarsh D, Wood S. Psychiatric aspects of destitution. In: Wing J, Haley A, eds. *Evaluating a community psychiatry service*. Oxford University Press, 1972.
5. Timms PW, Fry AH. Homelessness and mental illness. *Health Trends* 1989; **21**: 70–1.
6. George SL, Shanks NJ, Westlake L. Census of single homeless people in Sheffield. *British Medical Journal* 1991; **302**: 1387–9.
7. Reed R, Ramsden S, Marshall J, Ball J, O'Brien J, Flynn A, Elton N, El-Kabir D, Joseph P. Psychiatric morbidity and substance abuse among residents of a cold weather shelter. *British Medical Journal* 1992; **304**: 1028–9.
8. Lodge-Patch IC. Homeless men in London. 1. Demographic findings in a lodging house sample. *British Journal of Psychiatry* 1971; **118**: 313–7.
9. Priest RG. The homeless person and the psychiatric services: an Edinburgh study. *British Journal of Psychiatry* 1976; **128**: 128–36.
10. Marshall M. Collected and neglected: are Oxford hostels for the homeless filling up with disabled psychiatric patients? *British Medical Journal* 1989; **299**: 706–9.
11. Marshall EJ, Reed JL. Psychiatric morbidity in homeless women. *British Journal of Psychiatry* 1992; **160**: 761–9.
12. Adams CE, Duke PJ, Pantelis C, Barnes TRE. Homeless women: a prevalence study. Paper presented at the 36th annual meeting of the Society for Social Medicine, Nottingham, 1992.
13. Geddes J, Newton R, Bailey S, Young C, Freeman C, Priest R. Comparison of prevalence of schizophrenia among residents of hostels for homeless people in 1966 and 1992. *British Medical Journal* 1994; **308**: 816–9.
14. Hogg L, Marshall M. Can we measure need in the homeless mentally ill? Using the MRC needs for care assessment in hostels for the homeless. *Psychological Medicine* 1992; **22**: 1027–34.
15. Tantam D. High-risk groups: the homeless and ethnic minorities. *Current Opinion in Psychiatry* 1991; **4**: 295–303.
16. Breakey W, Fisher P, Kramer M, Neustadt G, Romanoski A, Ross A, Royall R, Stine O. Health and mental health problems of homeless men and women in Baltimore. *Journal of the American Medical Association* 1989; **262**: 1352–7.
17. Stark C, Scott J, Hill M. *A survey of the long-stay users of DSS resettlement units: a research report*. London: Department of Social Security, 1989.
18. Garety P, Toms P. Collected and neglected: are Oxford hostels for the homeless filling up with disabled psychiatric patients? *British Journal of Psychiatry* 1990; **157**: 269–72.
19. Lowry S. Concern for discharged mentally ill patients. *British*

Medical Journal 1989; **298**: 209–10.
20. Editorial. Homelessness. *Lancet* 1990; **ii**: 778–9.
21. Hall C. Ministers act on mental care. *Independent* 20 May 1992.
22. Bloomsbury Community Health Council. *Homeless and unhealthy in Bloomsbury.* 1989.
23. Marshall M, Gath D. What happens to homeless mentally ill people? Follow up of residents of Oxford hostels for the homeless. *British Medical Journal* 1992; **304**: 79–80.
24. Everton G. Disturbed face life on streets. *Oxford Mail* 16 September 1989.
25. Cohen N. Care in community leaving psychiatric patients homeless. *Independent* 23 October 1989.
26. Laidlaw S. Glasgow common lodging houses and the people living in them. Health and Welfare Committee of the Corporation of Glasgow, 1956.
27. Connelly J, Williams R. Schizophrenia among residents of hostels for homeless people. *British Medical Journal* 1994; **308**: 1572.
28. Borland A, McRae J, Lycan C. Outcomes of five years of continuous intensive case management. *Hospital and Community Psychiatry* 1989; **40**: 369–76.
29. Chamberlain R, Rapp C. A decade of case management: a methodological review of outcome research. *Community Mental Health Journal* 1991; **27**: 171–87.
30. Weller M, Tobiansky RI, Hollander D, Ibrahimi S. Psychosis and destitution at Christmas 1985–1988. *Lancet* 1989: **ii**: 1509–11.
31. Leff J. All the homeless people—where do they all come from? *British Medical Journal* 1993; **306**: 669–70.
32. Brugha TS. Support and personal relationships. In: Bennett DH, Freeman HL, eds. *Community psychiatry.* London: Churchill Livingstone, 1991: 115–61.
33. Joseph P, Bridgewater J, Ramsden S, El-Kabir D. A psychiatric clinic for the single homeless in a primary care setting in inner London. *Psychiatric Bulletin* 1990; **14**: 270–1.
34. Paykel ES. Contribution of life events to causation of psychiatric illness. *Psychological Medicine* 1978; **8**: 245–53.
35. Victor CR. Health status of the temporarily homeless population and residents of North West Thames region. *British Medical Journal* 1992; **305**: 387–91.
36. Bellack AS, Morrison RL, Wixted JT, Mueser KT. An analysis of social competence in schizophrenia. *British Journal of Psychiatry* 1990; **156**: 809–18.
37. Bughra D, Bullock R, Marshall J, Timms P. *Homelessness and mental illness.* Working party report on behalf of the Executive Committee of the General Psychiatry Section of the Royal College of Psychiatrists, 1991.
38. Leach J. Providing for the destitute. In: Wing JK, Olsen R, eds. *Community care for the mentally disabled.* Oxford: Oxford University Press, 1979: 90–105.
39. Ebringer E, Christie-Brown JRW. Social deprivation among short-stay psychiatric patients. *British Journal of Psychiatry* 1980; **131**: 46–52.
40. David AS. Insight and psychosis. *British Journal of Psychiatry* 1990; **156**: 798–808.

41. Murphy E. *After the asylums.* London: Faber & Faber, 1991.
42. Segal SP, Aviram U. *Community-based sheltered care: a study of community care and social integration.* New York: Wiley, 1977.
43. Thornicroft G, Halpern A. Legal landmark for community care of former psychiatric patients. *British Medical Journal* 1993; **307**: 248–50.
44. House of Commons Health Committee. *Better off in the community? The care of people who are seriously mentally ill.* Vol 1. London: HMSO, 1994.
45. Marshall M, Sharpe M. Untreated schizophrenia in hostels for the homeless: a cause for concern? *Bulletin of the Royal College of Psychiatrists* 1993; **17**: 16–8.
46. Mental Health Foundation. *Diversion, care and justice.* Conference documents. 1993.
47. Jones H. *Revolving doors: report of the Telethon inquiry into the relationship between mental health, homelessness and criminal justice.* London: NACRO, 1992.
48. Gunn J. Prisons, shelters and homeless men. *Psychiatric Quarterly* 1974; **48**: 505–12.

Chapter 6: Services for homeless people

1. Conway J, ed. *Prescription for Poor Health/The crisis for homeless families.* London Food Commission, Maternity Alliance, SHAC, Shelter, 1988.
2. Rogers CS. Health care of the homeless in the British NHS. *North Carolina Medical Journal* 1992; **53**: 228–34.
3. Foster P. *Access to welfare.* London: Macmillan, 1988.
4. Manchester Central Community Health Council. *Health care for homeless people.* Manchester Central CHC, 1980.
5. Williams S, Allen I. *Health care for single homeless people.* London: Policy Studies Institute, 1989.
6. Bayliss E, Logan P. *Primary health care for homeless single people in London—a strategic approach.* Single Homeless in London Health Sub-group, 1987.
7. Stern R, Stilwell B, Heuston J. *From the margins to the mainstream: collaboration in planning services with single homeless people.* West Lambeth Health Authority, 1989.
8. Fisher K, Collins J, eds. *Homelessness, health care and welfare provision.* London: Routledge, 1993.
9. Shiner M. *Adding insult to injury.* Unpublished MSc thesis, University of Surrey, 1991.
10. Powell PV. Qualitative assessment in the evaluation of the Edinburgh primary health care scheme for single homeless hostel dwellers. *Community Medicine* 1988; **10**(3): 185–96.
11. Scheuer M, Black ME, Victor C, Gill M, Benzeval M, Judge K. *Homelessness and the utilisation of acute hospital services in London.* King's Fund Institute. Occasional paper 4, 1991.
12. Clark C. 'Accessible, acceptable, appropriate'. *Health Service Journal* 11 March 1993.
13. Wake M, ed. *Housing and care needs of older homeless people.* Annual report. Arlington House, 1991.

14. Access to Health Project. *Models of good practice* (14 booklets). London: Access to Health, 1992.
15. Henwood M, Wistow G. *Hospital discharge and community care: early days.* Department of Health/Nuffield Institute for Health, 1993. *See also:* Workbook on hospital discharge. Department of Health, 1994.
16. NHS Management Executive. *General medical services to homeless people.* EL(92)27, 13 April 1992.
17. House of Commons Health Committee. *Better off in the community? The care of people who are seriously mentally ill.* First report (1993–4 session). Vol 1. London: HMSO, 1994.
18. Royal College of Psychiatrists. *Homelessness and mental illness.* Council report CR13. October 1991.
19. Shepherd A. Inside drug and alcohol misuse: struggling at the margins. *Community Care* 26 November 1992.
20. Connelly J, Kelleher C, Morton S, St James D, Roderick P. *Housing or homelessness: a public health perspective.* London: Faculty of Public Health Medicine, 1992.
21. Arnold P, Page D. *Housing and community care: bricks and mortar or foundation for action.* Report to the Major City Councils' Housing Group.
22. Arnold P, Page D, Bochel M, Brodhurst S. *Community care: the housing dimension.* York: Joseph Rowntree Foundation, 1994.
23. Departments of the Environment and Health. *Housing and community care.* Joint Circular. 10/92 (DoE), LAC(92)12 (DoH).
24. Randall G, Todd M. *In on the Act: CHAR's introductory guide to homelessness legislation and single people.* London: Campaign for Homeless and Rootless, 1993.
25. Smith SJ, McGuckin A, Hill S, Alexander A. *Housing provision for people with health problems and mobility difficulties.* Five reports available from Smith SJ, Department of Geography, University of Edinburgh. Summary available as *Housing research findings* No. 86. York: Joseph Rowntree Foundation, 1993.
26. Medical Campaign Project. *Vulnerability and community care.* London: MCP, 1992.
27. Prescott-Clarke P, Clemens S, Park A. *Routes into local authority housing: a study of local authority waiting lists and new tenancies.* Department of the Environment. London: HMSO, 1994.

Chapter 7: **Conclusions**

1. Report of a study group chaired by Sir Donald Acheson. *Primary health care in inner London.* London Health Planning Consortium, 1991.
2. Boyle S, Smaje C. *Primary health care in London: quantifying the challenge.* London: King's Fund, 1993.
3. Shanks N, Smith SJ. British public policy and the health of homeless people. *Policy and Politics* 1992; **20**: 35–46.
4. Connelly J, Kelleher C, Morton S, St James D, Roderick P. *Housing or homelessness: a public health perspective.* London: Faculty of Public Health Medicine, 1992.

Appendices

1. Great Chapel Street Medical Centre. Annual report, 1991–2.
2. Wytham Hall Sick Bay. Annual report, 1991–2.
3. HHELP East London Homeless Health Primary Care Team. Annual report, 1991–2.
4. Primary Health Care Project for Homeless People in Bristol. Avon FHSA. Half-year report, 1 April to 30 September 1992.
5. Leeds Health Care Team for the Homeless. Annual report, 1991–2.
6. Luther Street Centre, Oxford. Annual report, 1992–3.
7. Hanover Street Project. Annual report, 1992–3.
8. Petch H, Owens P. *The Bayswater Families Doctors Practice: a study of a mainstream primary health care service for homeless people.* CAIPE, LSE, 1992.
9. Chaplin J. Marylebone Health Centre: a unique approach to primary health care. *Community Health Action* 23, Spring 1992.
10. Stein T. The long goodbye. *Health Service Journal* 11 March 1993.

General bibliography

1. Collett D. *Health and homelessness* (in Oxford) *and an HIV/AIDS perception and behaviour study* (of 100 homeless people). Oxford Homeless Medical Fund, 1992.
2. Featherstone P, Ashmore C. Health surveillance project among single homeless men in Bristol. *Journal of the Royal College of General Practitioners* 1988; **38**: 353–5.
3. George SL, Shanks NJ, Westlake L. Census of single homeless people in Sheffield. *British Medical Journal* 1991; **302**: 1387–9.
4. Keating F, Klein O, Manning P, Ratcliff M. *The homelessness and mental health initiative: one year on.* London: Research and Development for Psychiatry.
5. Department of Health. *The care programme approach for people with a mental illness referred to the specialist psychiatric services.* Circular HC(90)23/LASSL(90)11.
6. North C, Ritchie J. *Factors influencing the implementation of the care programme approach.* Research study carried out for the Department of Health by Social and Community Care Planning Research. London: HMSO, 1993.
7. Hudson, B. Coming up roses. *Health Services Journal,* 3 September 1992.
8. Lelliott P, Sims A, Wing J. Who pays for community care? The same old question. *British Medical Journal* 1993; **307**: 991–4.
9. Access to Health Project. *Purchasing and poverty: a guide to commissioning health services for homeless people.* London: Access to Health 1992.
10. Access to Health & Medical Campaign Project. *Community care planning and homeless people.* London: Access & MCP, 1992.
11. Robbins D, ed. *Community care: findings from Department of Health funded research 1988–1992.* London: HMSO, 1993.
12. Royal College of General Practitioners. *Statement on homelessness and general practice.* March 1993.
13. Hatchett W. Taken by surprise. *Community Care* 5 July 1990.

Index